THE
LEADERS
WITHIN

THE
LEADERS
WITHIN

Engagement, Leadership Development, and Succession Planning

STEPHEN R. MASON | KATHRYN G. DIES
LARRY MORGAN

ACHE Management Series

Your board, staff, or clients may also benefit from this book's insight. For information on quantity discounts, contact the Health Administration Press Marketing Manager at (312) 424-9450.

This publication is intended to provide accurate and authoritative information in regard to the subject matter covered. It is sold, or otherwise provided, with the understanding that the publisher is not engaged in rendering professional services. If professional advice or other expert assistance is required, the services of a competent professional should be sought.

24   23   22   21   20   5   4   3   2   1

Library of Congress Cataloging-in-Publication Data
Names: Mason, Stephen R., author. | Dies, Kathryn G., author. | Morgan,
   Larry, 1943– author.
Title: The leaders within : engagement, leadership development, and
   succession planning / Stephen R. Mason, Kathryn G. Dies, Larry Morgan.
Description: Chicago, IL : Health Administration Press, [2020] | Series:
   HAP/ACHE management series
Identifiers: LCCN 2019019946 (print) | LCCN 2019022064 (ebook) | ISBN
   9781640551152 (print : alk. paper)
Subjects: LCSH: Executive succession. | Executive ability. | Leadership. |
   Health services administration.
Classification: LCC HD38.2 .M36795 2020 (print) | LCC HD38.2 (ebook) |
   DDC 658.4/092—dc23
LC record available at https://lccn.loc.gov/2019019946
LC ebook record available at https://lccn.loc.gov/2019022064

The paper used in this publication meets the minimum requirements of American National Standard for Information Sciences—Permanence of Paper for Printed Library Materials, ANSI Z39.48-1984. ∞ ™

Acquisitions editor: Jennette McClain; Project editor: Andrew Baumann; Cover designer: Brad Norr; Layout: PerfecType

Found an error or a typo? We want to know! Please e-mail it to hapbooks@ache.org, mentioning the book's title and putting "Book Error" in the subject line.

For photocopying and copyright information, please contact Copyright Clearance Center at www.copyright.com or at (978) 750-8400.

Health Administration Press
A division of the Foundation of the
   American College of Healthcare Executives
300 S. Riverside Plaza, Suite 1900
Chicago, IL 60606-6698
(312) 424-2800

This book is dedicated to Robert Dies—husband, father, and friend.
You are greatly missed.

Contents

Foreword

WHEN STEVE TOLD me that he was coauthoring a book on succession planning and leadership development, I knew I would say yes to the opportunity to write this foreword. My own career has benefited immensely from individuals who believed in planning for the future and building the skills of leadership at every level. It takes courage to be able to look ahead to your own departure from an organization and to train your successors while you are still on the job.

My own story begins with an unexpected health crisis and an empty CEO seat.

~

The board chair looked me straight in the eye and said, "Due to his illness, the CEO will be taking a sabbatical while his health improves. As the designated successor, you are now acting CEO."

The designated successor. I had held this position for nearly two years. In board meetings, I was casually referred to as the "hit-by-a-bus option." Now that option was in play, and I was going to be working closely with the board chair as interim CEO.

Fortunately, I was able to benefit from the foresight of the previous CEO. He was a good friend of mine who had invested time and energy in my leadership career over the course of two decades. He offered me mentorship, as well as increasingly significant management challenges, during those years. I was worried about his health and also concerned about my changing responsibilities. Although I felt reasonably prepared, I didn't know how much I didn't know.

I was also lucky that in my position as a stopgap CEO, I had the full support of the board chair, who had been an extremely sophisticated and experienced CEO in her own right. She and I worked together as a team to cultivate my executive skills and build my relationship with the board.

Over time, it became clear that the previous CEO would not be able to return, and the board began its search for a new CEO. Although I had held multiple executive-level positions in the health system, including acting CEO for the past six months, I was still a physician who was considered an outside-the-box choice to run this multihospital healthcare system. Nevertheless, my competencies and experience matched well with the board's strategic vision for the organization, and my credibility gave the board members enough confidence to offer me the job. To this day, I am certain that without the support and mentorship of the previous CEO, I would not have been given this opportunity.

There was just one catch. When the board members met with me to discuss my appointment as CEO, they stipulated that I would be required to be mentored by Ram Charan. Ram is an internationally known CEO, board consultant, and author who is often referred to as "the CEO whisperer." He has spent decades advising CEOs and boards all over the world, and our board wanted to give me every tool possible to be successful. At the time, I thought it was an interesting proposition. I had met Ram once before and thought he was a smart, well-connected man, but I wasn't clear on exactly what he would be teaching me.

Fast-forward several months to my first session with Ram. When I arrived at his hotel suite, he was on the phone with well-known CEOs whose names I could deduce from his end of the conversation. I felt humbled by his connections and his approach. Ram is a Harvard professor, and he carries that professorial style into all his work.

Immediately after his phone call concluded, he said to me, "Take out a piece of paper and write this down." I pulled out my pad and pen, ready to start taking notes. He went on, "If you want to be a successful CEO, there are three critical factors that you must know and do well: people, people, people. If you do those three things well, you will be successful. The organization you run is not about buildings, equipment, contracts, or strategies. It is about people, and you have to get that part right."

We spent the rest of the day deepening my understanding of people and talent. With the help of Ram's vast experience, I began to feel the way I always thought a competent CEO should. Ram's ongoing support, in addition to the support of the board chair and the previous CEO of my organization, gave me the foundation I needed for a positive start to my CEO career.

Over the next decade, our organization incorporated talent management, succession planning, leadership development, skill building, and other important people strategies. We executed some things extremely well and found other things to be extraordinarily difficult. As the organization fundamentally transformed from a fragmented aggregation of hospitals into a fully integrated, multistate health system, our outstanding people guided the strategy and led the way. People, people, people.

We started every board meeting with a conversation about leadership talent and succession planning for the entire senior leadership team, including my position. A board needs to lose only one CEO unexpectedly to become extremely interested in the succession planning process. In one of these conversations, I proposed a potential timeline for my retirement. This was a full five years before I ultimately retired, and because we had maintained ongoing discussions about the organization's leadership, this conversation was neither disruptive nor surprising.

Together, we committed to preparing two or three internal candidates who would interact broadly with the board, and we continued to discuss how these candidates might fit into the future vision of the organization. A supportive board can be invaluable to a CEO in selecting a successor. Each board member brings different experiences, an alternate perspective, and fresh eyes untainted by relationships or politics to the succession planning process.

Two years before the anticipated date of my retirement announcement, we had identified two strong internal candidates. I proposed to the board that these two leaders divide and share leadership of the company. Their success would be determined not only by each leader's independent performance but also by how well they collaborated and worked together as a team. My job was to help these individuals navigate any rough spots and continue to facilitate their leadership development. The two executives did an outstanding job working together and sharing responsibilities.

I announced my retirement 12 months before I left the organization. This gave the board plenty of time to assess the two internal candidates and to search for an external candidate if they felt that was necessary. The board selected one of the two candidates in four months, and I spent the next eight months staying out of the way.

This process gave the organization tremendous continuity with minimal disruption. Even the candidate who was not selected as CEO stayed on with the company because he knew how much he was valued. The new leadership team announced its strategies and initiatives and moved forward without missing a beat.

Planning for the succession of a CEO is a critical piece of the overall talent management strategy of an organization, but it is never the whole picture. The best succession planning programs address the leadership needs of the entire organization as it transforms to meet new market challenges. The success of a company depends on excellent leadership, management, and governance at every level.

The right people in management. The right people on the board. The right person as CEO. The right employees working for the organization. It's all about meshing competency, personal style, values, experience, and leadership with the strategies and mission of the organization. As my coach, Ram, told me many, many years ago, "If you get the people part right, you just might be a good CEO."

Steve and I have been friends and have moved in the same industry circles for many years. I greatly admire the succession planning and leadership development program that he and Dr. Dies have developed together. Their work is illustrative of the best qualities that leaders should embody. They are 100 percent dedicated to their cause, willing to adapt as circumstances change, and unafraid to admit and learn from their mistakes. Above all, they are helping each individual in the organization reach and express their full potential. People, people, people.

—John Koster, MD
CEO Emeritus
Providence St. Joseph Health

Preface

WE, THE AUTHORS of this book, worked for more than a decade to create, expand, and sustain a succession planning and leadership development program at a major health system. Steve had originally approached Kathie with an idea about the future of leadership in our organization, and that began a journey that led us to a legacy program. The program has grown beyond what we could ever have imagined ten years ago. We want to share that program with every organization that values its culture and the people who make it possible—the employees.

Our involvement in succession planning and leadership development represents decades of work in our collective careers. The knowledge we have gained over years of hiring and developing leaders, sometimes through trial and error, has refined the approach described in this book.

It is our hope that sharing these lessons will help you, the reader, broaden your view of what is possible for each member of your team, from the highest-level executive to the most junior new hire on staff. Our succession planning and leadership development program prototype can be adapted by an organization of any size to positively affect its leadership culture and strengthen its executive team. We pass on this information in the hope that it will benefit other organizations and inspire the individuals who work for them to become better leaders.

Acknowledgments

I AM INCREDIBLY grateful for the experiences I've had during my more than 35 years in a very rewarding industry, and to have had the privilege to serve and lead the growth and development of so many talented leaders over the years. I have visibly seen the immense changes that result when a group of people are dedicated and committed to an organization and an idea.

I particularly want to thank the entire board of directors for the BayCare Health System, especially Tom Whidden, Larry Morgan, and Bill Tapp, under whose chairmanships this book came to life. I wish to acknowledge Craig Brethauer, Kyle Barr, and Robert Garry for their support and leadership. I want to thank Tommy Inzina and his entire leadership team for their support and involvement in the success of BayCare's succession planning program. I owe a special acknowledgment to Kristen Sweeney, whose writing and editing skills brought great clarity and refinement to this book.

Finally, this book would not be possible without the love and support of my wife, Wanda, and daughter, Amanda.

—Steve

Having the opportunity to bring three decades of experience to life in the succession planning program of the BayCare Health System occurred thanks to the support received from the board of directors and senior leadership team, as Steve has acknowledged.

Additionally, the leadership development coaches who brought the training to life in the classroom were pivotal to the success of the program. Equally important, every leader who took on the role of coach for his or her direct reports demonstrated what leadership development is all about.

Lastly, the love and encouragement of my husband and partner in all things, Dr. Bob Dies, always kept me grounded and moving forward.

—Kathie

I would like to express my gratitude for the support I received from the BayCare board of directors and executive staff while I was chairman of the board. Under Steve Mason's leadership, BayCare experienced tremendous growth, expanding from a small community organization to one of the leading healthcare systems in the nation.

When the board of directors was faced with the pending retirement of our CEO, we suddenly realized we needed not only a succession plan for that position but also a formalized plan for all leadership positions in the organization. Under the direction of Kathie Dies, a thorough and comprehensive organizational structure was developed to provide continuous leadership for years to come. As I look at the ongoing growth and improvements in the BayCare organization today, I am proud to have been a small part of the endeavor that continues to serve our community's healthcare needs.

—Larry

Introduction

WHAT IS SUCCESSION PLANNING?

Succession planning is an ancient concept that dates to a time when societies operated under rigid social hierarchies and caste systems. Class and social status determined an individual's position in life and the role that individual was intended to play. For example, a shoemaker's son would prepare to replace his father as shoemaker, while the son or daughter of a reigning monarch would prepare for eventual ascension to the throne. One's role in life determined the kind of training one received.

Although children in many parts of the world today have more options available when choosing a career, the process of succession planning continues to live on in business. Like the family in earlier times, the company passes on valuable knowledge, providing novices with experience and teaching specific skills necessary to perform in the position one is destined to hold. In the modern corporation, succession planning is narrowly defined as creating a seamless way of transitioning the role of the senior-most executive from one individual to another. A broader view defines succession planning as a strategy to expand the reach of the company over the long term, creating a nimbler organizational design and effectively managing its political, economic, and business success.

The CEO (or other titled senior-most executive) of any organization is responsible for setting the vision and strategy that will consistently move the organization toward achieving its mission.

This responsibility requires making sure that the right talent and resources are available to meet every challenge that the organization may face. The CEO must continuously evaluate and reevaluate the alignment of the company's human talent with its strategic direction and performance goals.

From this point of view, succession planning becomes a strategy that is integral to an organization's survival. A strong succession planning process can reduce recruitment costs, create career development opportunities, reduce onboarding time, and ensure continuity with long-term organizational plans. Even more important is the cultural benefit that comes from demonstrating to employees that their hard work and commitment can lead to the acquisition of new skills and potential promotion. If you believe, as we do, that a strong culture is the lifeblood of every organization, then investment in your leaders is a critical step toward keeping your company alive.

Succession planning is often criticized for being expensive, and it is true that developing and training employees involves certain costs. It is also true that some of those employees may not be promoted and that others may ultimately leave the organization for a new job. One might therefore conclude that succession planning is an unwarranted expense because it prepares most employees to depart for positions with the competition. However, we have found that these assumptions do not correctly reflect the true value of succession planning. A company that is dedicated to the process not only achieves significant savings but also is strengthened in other ways. Succession planning offers the exciting opportunity to foster the growth and development of highly regarded employees, those who already understand the organization and its culture on a profound level.

Many organizations hire people from outside 80 percent of the time and hire internally only 20 percent of the time. The overall philosophy and strategy of this book is that this ratio should be reversed. You should aim to fill positions internally 80 percent of the time (and also strive to make sure internal candidates are the best people for the position 80 percent of the time). The talent pool in your organization, no matter its size, is one of your most valuable assets, and you can leverage it so that the most talented people inside the organization are available for promotion most of the time. Of course, the organization will occasionally need to search outside to fill unique roles that require a level of skill that is higher than what the internal candidate pool possesses, or if a new role has been created to address an important organizational strategy and no internal candidate currently possesses the talent or experience to perform that role.

WHAT IS LEADERSHIP DEVELOPMENT?

Whereas succession planning looks ahead to the role an employee may play in the future, leadership development focuses on improving that employee's skills in a current role. It is our belief that every employee—manager or nonmanager—can embody personal leadership while at work, in any role in the organization. Thus, developing leaders is about far more than ensuring that the futures of the top few spots in the company are secure. Leadership development gives the gifts of innovation and empowerment, helps employees think for themselves, and teaches them how to envision the world in which they want to live. An organization full of leaders benefits far more than the bottom line. Leadership improves and strengthens company culture, and it indirectly strengthens the families of those who work in the organization and even the community at large. A workforce of potential CEOs is one of the greatest assets an organization could ever hope to acquire.

SUCCESSION PLANNING VERSUS LEADERSHIP DEVELOPMENT

If you zoom the lens out far enough, you will see that both succession planning and leadership development are focused on the same goal:

developing talent from within to maintain organizational continuity. Is it possible to focus on a few individuals for succession planning and ignore an organization's broader leadership development? As a short-term solution, yes, but as a sustainable model for creating a pipeline of talent, absolutely not. You may be lucky enough to have a candidate who is ready to replace the CEO this time around, but that does not guarantee you will have candidates 10, 15, or even 20 years down the road who possess the skill set necessary to do the job. Looking at succession planning and leadership development as a single unit is critical because implementing one without the other is inefficient and will not produce measurable results that lead to confidence in the recruiting process. Although succession planning garners the most attention in a company, it is only part of the overarching theme of leadership development. In a sense, leadership development is succession planning on an organization-wide scale. It is preparing for the future—not just of a few key positions but of the company at large.

> I once worked for a man who told his board that nobody on his senior leadership team could replace him. A very seasoned corporate executive on the board challenged him, saying, "You don't know that to be true. It's not the job of your senior leadership team to upstage their boss." I never forgot that board member's confidence in our potential, in our ability to rise to the occasion when the time was right.
>
> —Steve

A TWO-TIERED APPROACH

We have created and implemented a simple, two-tiered framework to describe and develop the ideas of succession planning and leadership development (exhibit 0.1). Tier 1, traditional succession planning, emphasizes the development of candidates who could be

Exhibit 0.1: A Two-Tiered Approach to Succession Planning

Tier 1
Traditional
Succession Planning

- Includes a smaller pool of candidates with personalized development programs
- Identifies and improves specific competency gaps in leadership skills
- Prepares candidates to fill key leadership positions within five to seven years

Tier 2
Talent Pipeline

- Increases the depth of leadership development within the organization
- Takes a more broad-based approach to leadership skills
- Engages candidates not necessarily in leadership roles
- Enhances and improves candidates' skills in current roles
- Ensures long-term potential for key leadership positions

promoted to key leadership positions in the intermediate future. This tier identifies a relatively small number of candidates and works to improve specific gaps in each candidate's leadership abilities and competencies in preparation for key leadership roles five to seven years down the road.

Tier 2 is the talent pipeline aspect of the program, which seeks to increase the depth of leadership development training by incorporating candidates into the program earlier in their careers. Tier 2 typically evolves through several phases, expanding through the company from the top down over time. Its aim is to create a breadth and depth of talent that can eventually sustain Tier 1 long-term. Although the overall aims of Tier 1 focus on promotion and ascendancy, in actual implementation both Tier 1 and Tier 2 focus on enhancing candidates' skills and competencies to be maximally effective in their current roles as they prepare for the future.

Going forward, Tier 1 of the two-tiered approach will be referred to as *succession planning* and Tier 2 will be referred to more broadly as the *talent pipeline* or *leadership development*. Remember that Tier 1 is really a subset of Tier 2—in an organization, *all* leaders should receive leadership development. From the pipeline of individuals who receive leadership development, a limited number of candidates are eventually drawn into the succession planning program. Succession planning is thus elective, requiring referral into the program; leadership development is required of all leaders in an organization, whether they want to be promoted or merely want to learn to perform optimally in their current positions.

> If you focus only on the individuals you can process through succession planning, you've lost the opportunity to groom and grow all the other leaders in your organization. Then, when you have an unplanned vacancy, you're scrambling. That's what the talent pipeline is all about—developing people without the laser focus of where they might end up.
>
> —Kathie

When the desired outcome of an organization's culture is to seek first to promote from within, succession planning and leadership development must be fully integrated with one another. The aspect of assessment in succession planning and the establishment of development plans that address competency gaps best serve the organization when internal or coordinated internal and external candidates have the opportunity to engage in learning opportunities. Likewise, leadership development programs best serve the organization when the training offered is specifically linked to the organization's strategic goals.

Succession planning and leadership development are two manifestations of the same core principles: a commitment to company values, a desire to foster leadership potential, and a long-term vision for the organization's success. Succession planning, along with its companion, "talent management," is a specific component of overall leadership development. The initial focus is on the executive level (Tier 1), which comes with its own set of considerations for succession planning. Then, as leadership development becomes an organization-wide initiative, succession planning extends to include all leaders and potential leaders (Tier 2), subject to the modifications of operating at greater depth and scale.

In this book, we provide a comprehensive outline of both succession planning and leadership development, with the overarching caveat that these programs are meant to interact dynamically with one another in a way that adjusts to the changing environment of a given organization.

When you have finished reading this book, you will have learned the following:

- The three crucial roles in succession planning and leadership development (the Visionary, Architect, and Board Advocate), as well as the specific responsibilities of the individuals in each of those roles
- The specific benefits that organizations gain from integrating succession planning and leadership development programs, including benefits to the company's bottom line
- How to educate and inspire both the board and the executive team to secure organizational buy-in on succession planning and leadership development
- Why building a culture of leadership at all levels of a company is imperative for running a robust succession planning program
- How to create a dynamic succession planning and leadership development process that adjusts according to organizational strategic goals and establishes tiers of candidates as the program matures
- An effective method to identify potential candidates for succession planning and to assess their competency strengths and areas for development
- The step-by-step process for replacing key leaders in an organization while maintaining a high level of leadership continuity

- The nuts and bolts of designing a leadership development curriculum
- How to create an effective coaching environment to enhance the professional development of leaders throughout the organization

Establishing a succession planning and leadership development program requires focus, determination, and a little bit of grit. We believe that succession planning and leadership development are a vital part of any organization, but you shouldn't just take our word for it. For such programs to be effective, you need to understand what succession planning and leadership development can do for your organization and craft your goals, methods, and programs accordingly. Parts I–III (chapters 1–11) of this book focus primarily on establishing a succession planning program (Tier 1), and parts IV–V (chapters 12–22) examine the talent pipeline of leadership development (Tier 2).

We have identified four important reasons for implementing succession planning:

1. **To carry the company's vision into the future.** Succession planning and leadership development offer you the opportunity to strengthen the mission, vision, and values that make up your company culture. Developing and promoting internal candidates allows you to maintain greater organizational continuity during the turnover of high-level positions, such as president or CEO.

2. **To engage, retain, and promote candidates from within.** The greatest benefits from developing internal candidates are employee engagement and retention. You will gain lifelong employees and a reputation for being an organization that offers development opportunities, allowing you to consistently attract new talent. As you will see, this "mind-set of opportunity" has a cascading effect that affects employees at every level.

3. **To anticipate future changes and shifts.** An organization that is willing to invest in leadership development is an organization willing to confront the future head-on. The succession planning methods we recommend allow you to continually refine and redefine what the next generation of leadership will look like in your company and to stay well ahead of the curve when it comes to market changes in your industry.

4. **To avoid having many key leadership positions vacant at the same time.** Strategic planning and programming can prevent you from being blindsided if a significant percentage of your key leadership team retires or departs within a short period of time, leaving vacancies in the upper echelons of management. In chapter 5, we discuss how unanticipated turnover in even one key position can have significant financial repercussions for your company.

Before diving into your own organization's process, be sure you have clearly defined terms such as *company culture* and have set goals for employee retention and ratios of internal to external candidates that meet your specific parameters. We always recommend that this initial planning phase involve the governing body, which we discuss in more detail in chapter 5.

In the next few chapters, we address the elements of the initial succession planning process, which can be broken down into five major categories: who, what, when, where, and why.

PART I

Establishing Succession Planning and Leadership Development

CHAPTER 1

Valuing Succession Planning and Leadership Development: Why

INCORPORATING STRONG, THRIVING succession planning and leadership development programs into a large organization is a tremendous undertaking. The required investment of time, resources, and personnel is significant, which makes it imperative that the three key individuals involved—the Visionary, Architect, and Board Advocate—have a clear understanding of the value of implementing these programs. They should be able to clearly articulate *why* succession planning and leadership development are important based on their individual roles in the organization:

- **The Visionary's "why."** The Visionary's role is to paint a picture of the future and help everyone in the organization see it. One of the best ways to establish this future perspective is to put a succession planning program in place. A succession planning program clearly illustrates the organization's commitment to upward mobility and the growth of its team members, as well as an intention to be around for years to come. From the Visionary's perspective, a succession planning program helps build a staff of individuals who are dedicated to the organization and willing to work together to continue moving it forward. To be successful, the Visionary needs to commit to being the "messenger-in-chief" about succession planning and leadership development. He needs a clear, simple message about the long-term benefits these programs will provide to the organization.

- **The Architect's "why."** The Architect's role is to create a blueprint for bringing the Visionary's picture of the future to life. Her job is to design and implement the critical infrastructure that will be required to make succession planning and leadership development a consistent part of the company's culture. To the Architect, these programs add value because they promote skill building and personal growth at every level of the company. The Architect highlights how these programs make the organization more productive, creative, and collaborative—and better equipped to handle future challenges.

- **The Board Advocate's "why."** The Board Advocate's role is to maintain stability and longevity in the organization. Therefore, he is primarily concerned with how succession planning and leadership development can be used to smoothly transition high-level leadership positions from one individual to another and to avoid frequent or highly disruptive executive turnover. The Board Advocate also has a significant fiscal responsibility to the organization. As such, he values succession planning and leadership development as long-term investments that will save the company significant sums. The Board Advocate must be able to articulate these points to his fellow board members, whose approval and support are critical to building successful succession planning and leadership development programs.

Although the Visionary, Architect, and Board Advocate have slightly different perspectives on why succession planning and leadership development are important to an organization, their viewpoints overlap significantly. These programs offer an organization stability,

In our conceptualization of succession planning and leadership development programs, we, the authors—Steve, Kathie, and Larry—represent the Visionary, Architect, and Board Advocate, respectively. This book therefore refers to the Visionary as "he," the Architect as "she," and the Board Advocate as "he" for consistency throughout the text.

evidenced by higher employee retention; long-term financial savings; and smooth transitions of executive leadership positions. Stability also allows an organization to be more forward thinking, which is supported by the commitment to improve leadership skills at all levels of the organization as well as by the board's ability to understand how an investment in these programs is an investment in the organization's future. All three key individuals need to understand the complete picture of the value that succession planning and leadership development provide—although they may highlight or tailor certain elements of their message, depending on the audience.

Now that the value of succession planning and leadership development has been established, it is time to dive in and get started.

CHAPTER 2

Timing Succession Planning: When

THERE IS NO emergency strategy for succession planning. If you have an empty slot to fill and you aren't prepared to fill it internally, your only choice is to conduct an external search to find the right person for the job, which won't allow you to be selective in your choice. Nor will you have the time to spend cultivating an internal candidate who is a great fit but needs additional guidance. A vacant seat at the executive level affects day-to-day operations and can have a significant impact on the company's bottom line. Our two-tiered succession planning and leadership development program can prepare your organization for such unexpected leadership opportunities, which might otherwise have been emergencies.

So *when* should you begin succession planning? Right now—today. The preliminary planning and board education alone may require an entire year. And ideally, you want a minimum of five years' worth of data and development in place before you begin to consider internal candidates as replacements for key leadership positions. Assuming all your executives aren't planning to retire early or leave for another opportunity before age 65, you should anticipate that it will be approximately six years before you can put a mature succession planning program into action.

If you look at the first day of a new job as the first day of the job that you are going to invent for yourself, then you can see the value of succession planning led by leadership development. Success in any job is the ability of leaders to continuously reinvent themselves throughout the course of their careers by adjusting business strategies to the pace of the industry's evolution. To do this effectively, leaders needs to surround themselves with forward-thinking, creative, and highly trained people. The investment in leadership development produces significant cultural growth, promotes individual self-esteem, and prepares the organization for future leadership needs.

> It's the CEO's responsibility to spearhead succession planning, and he or she should start the very first day on the job.
>
> —Steve

With fresh perspective, the newly hired CEO should start thinking about developing a seamless plan for the organization, led by the most capable and prepared leaders possible, on the first day of a new job. Think about it this way: If the best practice in business is to begin the process of contract renewal with every customer on the day the first contract is signed, why wouldn't the same strategy apply to the succession planning and leadership development that are required to prepare leaders for the next level of growth? Taking this approach makes leadership development activity an organizational imperative.

Remember, succession planning is playing the long game, and this is where the real strategy comes into play. Who in your organization is willing to look as far forward as his or her own departure? Although long-term strategies may carry less urgency than the next big project that comes across your desk, the ability to clearly see an outcome that is still a decade away can make or break a company.

CHAPTER 3

Leading Succession Planning: Who

THE VISIONARY

Succession planning and leadership development typically start with the individual at the top of the organization, and ideally under the direct oversight of the board of directors. This individual—the Visionary—sees the future potential of the organization and its employees. He must be deeply invested in cultivating that potential and in supporting and elevating those around him. The task of lifting up others is a mighty one and requires the Visionary to be highly self-confident and not easily threatened by the success he helps create.

Being a leader, even an excellent leader, does not guarantee being a strong visionary for leadership development. For many CEOs, presidents, and founders, the idea of contemplating their inevitable departure and ultimate successor strikes a nerve. They have trouble admitting, even to themselves, that leaving the company is inevitable and that there will come a day when they no longer head into the office. Some leaders struggle with the notion that they are replaceable; as much as they wish for their company to succeed, they cannot imagine their organization actually carrying on without them. Thus, many leaders do not undertake the initiatives necessary to begin succession planning, and many organizations lack successful succession planning programs.

The Visionary is a person who can take on concepts as daunting as his own mortality. He doesn't pull rank or make exceptions for himself; rather, he participates in training alongside his employees. He is an individual who makes time in his own schedule to coach, guide, and mentor others. This is the style of leadership that is needed for an effective succession planning process.

As a leader, the Visionary doesn't just envision a world where a succession planning program runs smoothly for his organization; he is also responsible for sustaining this vision for the individuals in the succession planning program. If his dream becomes a reality, all company employees will see themselves as potential leaders in the workplace, and hopefully as leaders in their families and communities as well. Sustaining a vision for others is about inspiration, not motivation; people will motivate themselves if they feel inspired. The Visionary's job is to hold up a picture of what is possible and then inspire his team members to create and step into that possibility for themselves.

The Visionary must be able to see the potential in others, regardless of how undeveloped that potential may currently be. Leadership is not innate from birth; rather, individuals need to be fostered to develop leadership skills. Leadership development is ultimately about helping and empowering people and creating the conditions for a switch to flip inside their brains. When the switch flips, they boldly confront challenges or new opportunities and proclaim, "Yes, I could do that."

The Visionary has a big job and a long road ahead. The good news is that he doesn't have to do it alone. A partner can take on the responsibility of creating and shaping the logistics, workflow, and operational mechanisms of a succession planning program, building out his vision from top to bottom. The Visionary paints in broad brushstrokes, but someone else fills in the details—the Architect.

THE ARCHITECT

The second major player in this process, the Architect, is charged with filling in the details: drawing up the blueprints, breaking the ground, and overseeing the actual construction of a succession planning and leadership development program. She works closely with the Visionary to execute what he sees, but she has unique skills and qualifications that both complement and foil the Visionary.

Whereas the Visionary supplies the *why* of succession planning and leadership development, the Architect figures out *how* these aims will be achieved and *what* the complete program structure will look like. While the Visionary will continue in his previous role in the organization as CEO or president, the Architect will hold a new position expressly dedicated to succession planning and leadership development. She is ultimately the epicenter of any mature succession planning and leadership development program.

As mentioned, the Architect works to fill in the Visionary's broad strokes. Just how broad those strokes start out depends on the dynamic between these two. The Visionary needs to provide the guiding principles and the anticipated outcomes of the process, and the Architect's job is to convert those big ideas into seamless, fluid, and functioning programs.

In summary, the Visionary and the Architect have different backgrounds, skill sets, and qualifications for their roles. The Visionary is focused on the big picture of how to achieve the organizational success that has been forecast. The Architect's position is dedicated to succession planning and leadership development and to providing trained employees who are vital for meeting the organization's key goals.

THE BOARD ADVOCATE

Even if the Visionary and the Architect can technically execute the mechanics of succession planning and leadership development programs on their own, they need board support to move forward and embed a culture of leadership into the organization's DNA (although the extent to which the board exerts control depends on the company's structure). This support comes from the third key figure in the process—the Board Advocate.

The Board Advocate acts as a liaison between the Visionary and Architect duo and the board itself. Regardless of his position on the board, the Board Advocate can expect to take a leadership role with respect to educating his fellow board members and enrolling their support for the establishment and growth of these programs.

QUALIFICATIONS AND REQUIREMENTS

What the Visionary Needs

The Visionary is ideally the CEO, president, or founder of the organization. He is the one who recognizes the need for succession planning and jump-starts the process. He not only provides critical momentum toward obtaining board approval for the program but also serves as the prime example of commitment to leadership development and to a graceful succession transition when he retires. It is vital that the Visionary fully embrace the program, including attending workshops, participating in team-building exercises, and completing work assigned by his coach. Otherwise, the program is all but guaranteed to fail. Whatever is required, the Visionary must be prepared to do it, being mindful that he is leading by example for every member of his organization.

What the Architect Needs

Whereas the Visionary is defined more by his role in the organization and the part he plays in initiating the succession planning process, the Architect's qualifications are much more specific. To fully implement a succession planning and leadership development program, the Architect needs a background in executive coaching and/or organizational development. Training in both is ideal, and an Architect with a background in organizational development can certainly pursue an executive coaching certification while establishing the succession planning program. Although her role may not initially be a full-time position, you may wish to hire a full-time employee in anticipation of the role's future expansion. Early on, this full-time employee could cross over to do some human resources (HR) work, as the HR department is likely to be the best match for her skill set. If your program is successful, however, you can anticipate that the Architect will eventually move away from HR work and begin leading a full-time staff of her own.

Expertise in executive coaching and organizational development allows the Architect to lay out a framework for succession planning and leadership development that can scale in size to accommodate a company of hundreds or perhaps thousands of employees. To do so effectively, she must understand the logistics necessary for the successful implementation of a succession planning program. As you will see, coaching is an integral part of leadership development; as an executive coach, the Architect may not only directly coach high-level executives but also train other leaders on how to coach their direct reports. She can step in when these leaders are having difficulties and course-correct their approaches as necessary.

The Architect is also responsible for selecting, implementing, administering, and interpreting various psychological and personality assessments as part of the succession planning program's candidate evaluation process. An executive coaching and organizational development background should provide her with a thorough working knowledge of these assessments and allow her to use those that are most appropriate to the company's specific needs.

Training in psychology also can be useful to the Architect, although it is not as critical as training in executive coaching or organizational development. A background in psychology may enable the Architect to identify when succession planning candidates need additional resources or outside help.

The Architect must be flexible and willing to embrace the dynamic nature of the succession planning and leadership development process, allowing her to adjust as the competency demands of the organization's leaders change over time. A program that evolves with its leaders is a program with great potential for making a lasting impact on the organization.

Finally, it is important that the Architect have strong competency for leadership. If the program is successful, she will eventually lead a team dedicated to the program and will need to effectively manage and inspire those individuals.

You might be wondering if the Architect has to be an employee of the organization or if it would be more effective to hire the Architect directly from a consulting company. In our opinion, having an Architect as a full-time staff member means you have an individual who has a deep understanding of your company's culture that most consultants simply cannot match. Working with people is significantly easier when you have cultivated ongoing relationships with them and have an office down the hall.

Although they can be of value to a company, consultants may not be the best solution for several other reasons. They can be perceived as outsiders and not accepted as credible members of the organization by existing employees, who tend to view consultants' work as just the latest in a series of pet projects undertaken by the organization. Consultant fees can be high and may not scale well when you are looking at deeply embedding succession planning and leadership development in an organization. The fees for external consulting, including assessment and coaching, may be justifiable for a handful of key company leaders, but less so for 150 individuals, and certainly not for a program that includes 1,000 employees or more. Many succession planning programs focus on providing for only the top three or four positions in the company as a way of managing expensive consulting costs and meeting the minimum expectations of good governance, but this is a short-term, stopgap measure and does not provide a talent pipeline to secure the organization's long-term future—nor does it offer the advantages of hiring an in-house Architect.

In certain cases, the Visionary may need to use a consultant for direction when an internal Architect is not readily identifiable. The consultation in such instances should be time limited, with a focus on helping the Visionary outline leadership development and succession planning to gain support from the organization's board and its executive leadership. A consultant may also assist in identifying candidates who have the requisite skills to take on the role of Architect long-term.

The Architect is responsible for building relationships across the organization. She continually monitors candidates' progress and checks in with coaches. When you fuse succession planning with leadership development, you need an Architect who is immersed in the company's values. This allows her to change and develop the direction of the program as needed to meet the organization's goals and to provide continuity for and respond quickly to candidates' needs. The Architect should be sensitive to the nature and timing of requests from employees, such as asking managers to allow their direct reports to take time away from work for leadership training. An internal Architect understands the totality of the organization and how all the pieces fit together, and she recognizes that succession planning and leadership development are only one piece of the puzzle (albeit a very important one).

> We had an individual in our succession planning program who was being considered for a key leadership role and needed to enhance presentation skills. The individual's coach reached out to me to request some additional work around the full range of competencies involved in making presentations. I started working with this individual directly, and we were able to laser-focus on the areas that needed the most improvement. When the assigned coach and the Architect work closely together, additional competency gaps can be identified early on and effectively addressed.
>
> —Kathie

What the Board Advocate Needs

In addition to the technical requirement that the Board Advocate be a sitting member on the organization's board, this individual's other qualifications primarily relate to values and a willingness to commit. He must be passionate about the organization's mission, able and ready to play a significant leadership role, and dedicated to spending the extra time it may take to learn about the subject matter.

> I can't tell you how many days I spent at educational seminars to improve my knowledge of the healthcare field.
>
> —Larry

The Board Advocate does not necessarily need to have a background in the organization's industry. In fact, board members are often chosen for their external expertise, which allows them to bring a fresh perspective to the workings of the organization.

Above all, the Board Advocate should be an individual willing to learn and collaborate. He will have valuable opinions and insights to offer throughout the process, but he likely will not be an expert in building out a leadership development program. Therefore, he must be open to further education and must listen closely to the Visionary's and Architect's opinions and advice.

> When I first joined up with the organization that would become BayCare, I was asked to bring my knowledge as a business owner. I looked at the company's challenges and thought I had things figured out pretty quickly, until I realized that 90 percent of the things I wanted to do weren't permitted in the healthcare world!
>
> —Larry

CHAPTER 4

Determining Succession Planning Needs: What

CREATING A ROAD MAP

Once your Visionary and Architect are in place, the next step is to map out the terrain of your organization's future. What do the next five years look like? How about the next ten years? Which key leaders will likely still be part of the company, and which ones will be replaced by somebody new?

Before you can create this map, you must first determine which roles you consider to be key leadership positions and would therefore like to account for in a succession planning program. In smaller organizations, this may be the entire leadership team; in larger companies, it may include only the first few tiers of executives. The easiest way to complete this initial task is to use your company's current organizational chart.

For the model in this book, we use six tiers of leadership, which we have divided into five levels (A–E; see exhibit 4.1). A candidate's level determines whether he or she is eligible to join the succession planning program. The levels also differentiate some factors of an individual's leadership development, including the particulars of that individual's curriculum and additional resources that may be offered. (See chapter 15 for more information on differentiated leadership tracks.) A recurring theme throughout this book is our

Exhibit 4.1: Five Levels of Leadership

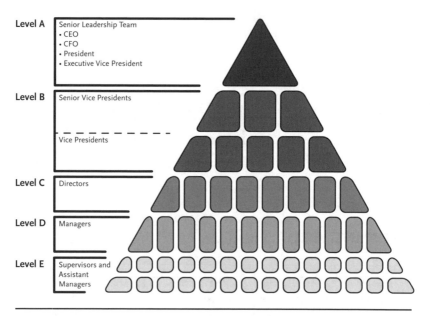

Level A — Senior Leadership Team
- CEO
- CFO
- President
- Executive Vice President

Level B — Senior Vice Presidents

Vice Presidents

Level C — Directors

Level D — Managers

Level E — Supervisors and Assistant Managers

wholehearted belief in leadership development for every leader in an organization, including all individuals with recognized leadership potential.

The structure of your company may differ from our example. If so, you can adapt our five-level model to match your organization's own leadership structure. Both succession planning and leadership development roll out in phases, and as you read the rest of this book it will be helpful to understand how these levels of leadership correspond to those of your organization.

Once you have created your corresponding organizational chart, determine what level of leadership you would like to account for in succession planning. If you want to include levels A and B, draw a horizontal line across your chart just below level B. All positions above the line are considered key leadership; all positions below the line may be added as you scale leadership development. When you create your first succession planning map, you will include only individuals in levels A and B. These positions are the most important to succession planning, because replacing the individuals who currently occupy these roles could have a significant impact on the organization. Including candidates at levels C and D will become the priority in the next phase of program development.

Although the individuals in leadership positions that fell directly below the line are not the first focus for succession planning, they are often part of the succession planning program. In general, level C candidates should be included in succession planning so they can be prepared to ascend to level B positions, and eventually to level A roles. You can see how the need for leadership development in the succession planning process is critical as it extends to include individuals in level D roles who may replace level C leaders. In this hypothetical model, level E individuals are not eligible for succession planning until they are promoted to a level D position, but as leaders in the organization, they should receive leadership development regardless of whether they are included in succession planning.

Once you have drawn your horizontal line and identified which positions you would like to account for, we recommend creating a projection of potential succession planning needs. This visual representation should show all of your key leadership positions, as well as the anticipated retirement dates for the individuals currently in those roles. The succession planning projection not only gives a clear picture of the trajectory of the company but will also be a persuasive element when it comes time to propose the succession planning program to your company's board (discussed in chapter 5).

Next, set a baseline departure age. This is the average age at which you expect your key leaders to retire. In the sample projection in exhibit 4.2, we've set the anticipated departure age at 67. Organizations that experience high employee retention will find that this example makes sense for them. It assumes that most key leaders who are within ten years of retirement are going to stay with the company rather than elect to change jobs at age 60 or 62. If your industry standard is that executives retire at age 60 or change positions every seven to ten years regardless of age, you might set

Exhibit 4.2: Sample Succession Planning Projection

Succession Planning Projection

Title	Age	2015	2016	2017	2018	2019	2020	2021	2022	2023	Age 67
President, CEO	67	67									2015
Executive Vice President, CFO	47										2035
Executive Vice President, Hospital President	53										2029
Executive Vice President, Medical Staff Relations	59									67	2023
Vice President, Laboratory Services	57										2025
Vice President, Team Resources (HR)	64				67						2018
Vice President, Finance	63					67					2019
Vice President, General Counsel	55										2027
Senior Vice President, Information Services	57										2025
Vice President, Central Business Services	58										2024
Vice President, Imaging and Ambulatory Surgery	53										2029
Vice President, Behavioral Health	63					67					2019
Vice President, Marketing and Communications	57										2025
Vice President, Medical Affairs	66		67								2016
Vice President, Chief Nursing Executive	54										2028
Vice President, Financial Services	60								67		2022
Vice President, Philanthropic Foundation	50										2032
Vice President, Operations	67	67									2015
Vice President, Medical Affairs	60								67		2022

your departure age differently. Once you have set your departure age, you are ready to create your succession planning projection.

Using your projection, you can get a clear visual picture of who, among your current leaders, can be expected to retire within five and ten years. You may find that the five-year projections look good, but the ten-year retirement forecast is potentially devastating to your organization. However, by preparing now for the possibility of having a significant number of vacant positions in the organization at the same time, you can avoid a possible crisis.

In addition to your succession planning projection, consider looking at your organization's historical data for replacing key leaders. How often do you hire internally, and how often do you go outside to fill executive roles?

When we looked at the current state of BayCare using a similar succession planning projection and examined our historical hiring data, we noticed two things. First, a number of leaders were expected to retire within the next decade; therefore, we would be facing significant vacancies in our key leadership. Second, we had historically replaced only 20 percent of our leadership positions with internal candidates and were hiring outside the organization about 80 percent of the time.

What we saw, when we looked at our succession planning projection, was a possible long-term recipe for disaster. The kind of large-scale leadership replacement we would have to confront in the next decade could make it extremely difficult for the company to maintain daily operational continuity. We faced a high number of costly candidate searches, as well as the economic impact that almost inevitably results from replacing key leaders. Furthermore, we were sending our employees a message that very few advancement opportunities were available to them, and we saw that this message threatened the company culture of engagement we had been working so hard to create and maintain. Once we understood how precarious the future of our organization could potentially be, we were determined to move forward, swiftly and effectively, with the succession planning program.

CRAFTING THE SUCCESSION PLANNING PROGRAM

This chapter intentionally appears before our discussion of presenting succession planning to the company's board because the Visionary and Architect must work together to flesh out the succession planning program before presenting it to the organization's governing body. If the program planning is not fully visualized, it will likely never come to fruition. Although nearly all organizations and leaders think succession planning is a good idea, for many companies it remains a good idea that is never put into practice. Organizations frequently consider succession planning a low-priority item that is allocated scant resources and not given the opportunity to flourish. Anticipating the full needs of the program before facing your board will give both you and your succession planning program a much greater chance of success.

The most rudimentary succession planning program might involve simply creating and interpreting a succession planning projection and then anticipating extensive candidate searches to replace a few high-level positions. In our view, however, succession planning and leadership development go hand in hand. Truly impactful succession planning enables employees to rise through the ranks via a talent pipeline, and it requires looking inside the company first. A strong succession planning program will always be paired with leadership development to prepare internal candidates for long-term career trajectories with plenty of opportunities to ascend to the next level. That said, the timing of the leadership development aspect of the program is variable. You may find, as we did, that by the time you begin crafting the succession planning program, you already have a foundational leadership development program in place. Hence, even in the early stages, our succession planning guidelines assumed the program would be supplemented by leadership development; this was particularly important for level B and level C executives who, with some development, might be positioned to take over level A roles in the not-too-distant future.

What follows are the foundations of a successful succession planning program. This overview will provide you with enough general structure and operational information to begin creating a succession planning program of your own. We talk briefly about leadership development here, but we address the talent pipeline of leadership development specifically in part IV. You will find additional details about the execution of both succession planning and leadership development in part V, "Nuts and Bolts."

Referral to the Program

The first step in planning the succession planning program is to determine how a candidate will be selected for entry into the program. This could be done on a self-referral (volunteer) basis, although this method is likely to make the program quite large rather quickly. Program entry could be based on a referral from the candidate's direct supervisor, which is the method we have chosen to employ and strongly recommend, or referrals could be solicited from only certain individuals, such as leaders at levels A and B. You could also opt for a hybrid program, where a self-referral is combined with the pledged support of a candidate's supervisor.

Assessment Battery

The assessment battery is a series of tests that address personality type, leadership style, relationships with others, and leadership competencies. The Architect will oversee the selection and subsequent administration of these assessments, which should cover the areas of intrapersonal and interpersonal characteristics, as well as emotional intelligence. You should also include a 360-degree assessment, which looks at hard skills such as financial acumen, critical thinking, and seasoned judgment in addition to some of the softer relational skills. A 360-degree assessment should include 20–25 competencies and solicit feedback from the candidate and his or her boss, direct reports, peers, and others. We recommend administering the battery of leadership assessments after an individual has been referred to the succession planning program.

Some organizations screen candidates for admittance to the succession planning program by requiring them to complete one or more leadership assessments. We discourage this practice of screening out candidates, for two reasons. First, the examinations can be costly, especially as a screening tool. Second, you want to show your referring managers that you value their opinions, and you want to show your referred candidates that you believe in their potential. If a candidate has been referred to and makes the commitment to succession planning, you should likewise accept the responsibility for nurturing his or her growth. If you do not screen out candidates, you can be sure every assessment you give is a worthwhile investment in a candidate's future.

Program Structure

The program structure is where you describe what the process of succession planning will look like on a daily basis. It clarifies the expectations, goals, and markers of success—not only to the board as they debate the merits of implementing your program but also to the eventual participants in the program. The succession planning and leadership development programs will each have a separate structure. In general, leadership development will be a more established curriculum, whereas succession planning will be highly individualized and tailored to the candidate's needs. The strongest programs will contain a mix of group training courses, private and group coaching sessions, outside resources as required, and some degree of external assignments. (We will discuss how these elements work together in both succession planning and leadership development in later chapters.) The Architect is responsible for creating the structure of each program, and she (and eventually her team) will lead the execution of each as well, including facilitating group programs, training and following up with coaches, handling any issues that may arise, and creating a system of ongoing data collection and feedback.

> Although succession planning programs are governed by a set of general rules, it's vital to make every program as specific to the individual company as possible. Each person on the management team brings a unique set of skills to their position that needs to be accounted for.
>
> —Kathie

CHAPTER 5

Getting the Board on Board: Where (It Comes Together)

ONCE THE VISIONARY and the Architect have created the program structure and developed the strategy for succession planning, good governance practices dictate that educating the board on the importance of leadership development and succession planning becomes a high priority. The technical purpose, organizational design, and mission of your organization may vary greatly from ours, but the underlying assumption we make is that the senior leadership and board of any company want to see continuous high performance and success throughout the life of the organization. To convince your board to support succession planning and leadership development at an organization-wide level, you will need to convey how these programs can accomplish those aims.

Because we felt it was important for our board members to understand the philosophy behind succession planning and leadership development, we at BayCare spent nearly a year educating them on the strategic advantages of establishing and operating these programs, emphasizing how important the board's buy-in was to the success of the process. We invested time and resources in putting together presentations, engaging in conversations, and being available for questions at every point throughout this period.

One practical reason boards often avoid talking about succession planning is that it can be an uncomfortable topic of conversation.

Board members feel awkward asking a CEO or vice president to step out of the room while they discuss the future of her position, and it can be equally awkward for her to remain and be part of the dialogue. Your organization can alleviate the anxiety around the succession planning conversation by making it a regular agenda item, discussed as an ongoing part of your adopted strategies. Doing so not only helps normalize the topic for executives and board members alike but also ensures that succession planning remains an ongoing, high-priority issue for your company.

The board may also feel troubled about succession planning when a leader who is excelling in his current role wants to be considered for the next level of leadership. This situation can arise when the succession planning process is looking at individuals in key leadership roles who have already contributed significantly to the organization's growth in their current roles. A significant mind-set adjustment goes along with endorsing a succession planning program: The board must realize that although the organization may be losing the skill sets of an individual in a certain role, it will be retaining a stellar leader by supporting his development for a new, more challenging role. Similarly, several individuals will be considered for each role in the early stages of the succession planning process, but only one of those individuals will advance. Yet, during the process, the organization will have had the advantage of growing the skills of all of the candidates throughout the development process.

When it is time to present your succession planning program to the board, clearly outline the following benefits and advantages:

- **Organizational continuity.** Every company wants a smooth, seamless transition from one CEO to the next. In a best-case scenario, succession planning provides this easy transition by identifying an internal candidate who has been receiving leadership development and is thoroughly prepared to take over the role. This candidate is already familiar with the day-to-day operations of the company. She knows where to find the conference rooms and how to log in to the e-mail system. These considerations may seem minor and temporary, but they eat into the time and energy of a new executive. Additionally, an internal succession planning candidate will have been preparing for the specific challenges of a new role for the past 6–18 months and will have had the opportunity to observe and work closely with the current CEO, giving her a real sense of what the position entails.

- **Preservation of company culture.** Aside from maintaining smooth daily operations and minimizing the technical onboarding process, the board should consider the advantages that an internal candidate offers with respect to preserving company culture. Many (though not all) organizations today spend a significant amount of energy on developing the company's mission, vision, and core values—that is, the company culture. Tremendous effort is devoted to infusing these ideas from the top to the bottom of the organization, so that each employee not only understands the company culture but also embraces and fully lives it. In this way, the company culture becomes a part of the organization's DNA.

   An external hire will require additional time to fully understand and integrate into your company culture. He may agree with the mission, vision, and values in theory, but his actions may not reflect alignment with these ideas. Moreover, he may not agree with all of the values. No amount of rigorous interviewing can fully predict an individual's behavior once he enters the workplace. The process of hiring an external candidate is simply no match for the daily observation of internal candidates in a succession planning program, where these candidates are coached and trained specifically in accordance with the company culture.

- **Cascading effect.** We discussed in the introduction that employee retention is a huge motivator for organizations to institute succession planning and leadership development programs. When a key leadership position is filled by an individual who already works for the company, employee retention extends beyond that individual. If an executive at level C ascends to a position at level B, there is now an open spot in level C management. A candidate at level D will likely be prepared to take over that position, leaving an opportunity at level D for a leader from level E to step into, and so on. Filling one position internally thus creates a sequence of other available roles. In other words, internal promotions lead to a cascading effect throughout the company. Employees see this opportunity for growth and, in turn, work harder to become better leaders. A successful succession planning program increases employee retention and improves job satisfaction throughout an entire organization. Part IV of this book provides a thorough example of the cascading effect that promotion through succession planning can have on an organization.

- **Ability to plan ahead.** Even if you determine that a position cannot be filled by promoting an internal candidate, the tools of succession planning can still prepare an organization for the departure of key leaders. Monies can be allocated in advance to a budget for an external search. Arrangements can be made for other leaders to cover certain vital responsibilities of the departing executive until the position has been filled. Occasionally, the role of a key leader needs to be reimagined or redefined because of shifts in the organization or industry. Succession planning allows your company to anticipate those changes so that when the time comes for hiring, even externally, you are crystal clear as to the specific qualifications that the next candidate must possess.
- **Financial repercussions.** Although you may have to spend time educating your board members on the importance of concepts such as the cascading effect of

internal promotions and the maintenance of company culture, you will likely find them eager and ready to discuss the financial repercussions of succession planning. Succession planning reduces an organization's costs in two main ways, which you should highlight to the board as you move forward with your program.

First, you save the company costly searches for external candidates. When a high-level executive is hired externally, the placement or executive search firm involved will collect a hefty fee—generally the equivalent of 30 percent of the new individual's salary. If you think about the salaries for the top five executives in your company, the amount of this finder's fee alone can easily be tens of thousands, and often hundreds of thousands, of dollars. Although this is the single largest expenditure when hiring an outside candidate, the process entails other costs as well.

Beyond agency fees, your organization must pay the travel expenses of all external candidates during the interview process, including airfare, hotel stays, and local transportation. Once a candidate has been selected, you will also be expected to pay for his or her relocation. Occasionally, an organization will get lucky and hire a local external candidate, but the higher up the ladder you go, the less likely this outcome becomes. When presenting to your board, try to pull numbers directly from your organization's own history. How much did you spend on your last candidate search? You should be able to easily demonstrate that by reducing the number of external candidates, you will be saving significant sums of money.

The second way succession planning reduces an organization's costs is more difficult to quantify, but it has important implications. When an external candidate enters a high-level position in a company, it takes him much longer to get up to speed than an internal candidate. A change in CEO, for example, disrupts the flow of business and alters social dynamics, but the dust will settle much faster with an internal candidate who already has a firm grasp on the company's values and culture and the course of daily operations.

The costs of such a change have historically been a challenge to pin down, and for that reason they are largely ignored when boards look at succession planning programs. However, Favaro, Karlsson, and Neilson (2015) measured these concerns and found they carried a hefty price tag—$112 billion, to be exact. Their research showed that an organization's financial performance is likely to decrease in the year before and the year after a CEO turnover. Although this finding includes turnovers involving both internal and external replacements, the authors concluded that companies without planned turnovers suffer much more than organizations with strong succession planning. The strongest succession planning stems from leadership development that guides and shapes leaders within the company.

In terms of new expenditures, succession planning will add the cost of the salaries for the Architect and her eventual team, as well as the cost of the assessment battery for each candidate. Aside from a small leadership development team on staff, the coaches in your organization will be your own employees, who will also receive ongoing leadership development, coaching, and mentoring. In our experience, these are salaried individuals whose performance has in no way suffered by dedicating a few hours each month to focus on the development of their own careers and the careers of their direct reports.

In fact, the skills taught in a succession planning program make leaders more effective and better able to deal with conflict when it arises. They experience less stress and have a better work–life balance. It is difficult to quantify these benefits with a number, but we firmly believe that these individuals add positive value to the organization, including to its bottom line. Taking all factors into consideration, you can easily demonstrate to your board that the long-term savings generated by succession planning will far exceed the expenses.

During this process, the Board Advocate will help the Visionary and the Architect offer the strongest evidence possible in favor of creating a succession planning and leadership development program. A company's board considers its role to be focusing on current leadership needs and maintaining the stability of the organization. Fortunately, it is easy to illustrate how succession planning and leadership development help the board achieve these goals. Ideally, the Board Advocate has already offered his support to the Visionary and Architect and is clearly convinced of the value of this invest-ment in the organization; therefore, together, this trio can work to persuade the rest of the board members. At its core, the best strategy is to show the board where the gaps are in organizational efficiency and strategy, and then offer solutions for filling in those gaps.

> As the Board Advocate, I was an easy sell on succession planning from day one. Steve and Kathie made it apparent that we had some voids in planning for the future of our leadership team, and they provided evidence that we needed a long-term plan for resolving these problems.
>
> —Larry

It is critical during this period that the Visionary sustain a clear picture of the organization's future and that the Architect offer practical solutions for making the vision a reality. Without the Visionary, the board will not grasp the level of organization-wide commitment necessary to implement the program. Without the Architect, the board will consider the vision an idealistic pipe dream. Finally, the hope is that the board is composed of smart, dedicated, and successful individuals who see the value of investing in the organization's long-term future.

> Our board did a cost analysis of the succession planning program, and our final conclusion was that we couldn't afford *not* to do it.
>
> —Larry

If the organization lacks a Visionary to drive the succession planning and leadership development process, the Board Advocate is in a difficult position because he is not the leader of the organization. It is highly unlikely that a program of this nature could be successfully implemented with a board member in the Visionary role. On the other hand, a lack of vision from an organization's executive leadership may indicate that some kind of board-driven, high-level leadership change is necessary (making succession planning all the more valuable).

If succession planning is in place when an organization gets a new CEO, that CEO should be immediately admitted into the succession planning program. Any candidate should be well vetted to ensure that he or she is comfortable discussing succession planning, both on a personal and on an organizational level.

Case Study

As a large healthcare organization, BayCare's decision to launch a succession planning program was a marked change from its history of hiring organizational leaders externally 80 percent of the time and promoting from within 20 percent of the time. The magnitude of this change required educating the board and executive leadership on the process that was to unfold—a

→

process that could not be rushed. An initial presentation to the board brought up numerous questions:

- How would the succession planning program affect the perception of current leaders?
- What were the repercussions of developing potential candidates internally and then losing some of them to other organizations?
- What was the possibility that strong current leaders might be lost to other roles in the organization?
- How could the gaps in organizational leadership and the personal professional gaps of individual leaders be determined?

The initial step was to take the time necessary to respond to individual concerns and to fully outline the process of succession planning. Then, benefits of the succession planning process were identified that outweighed the concerns about the impact the change would have on hiring processes.

The goal was to help the executive leadership team adopt the vision of a succession planning process that would benefit them both personally and professionally as leaders of their direct reports. Another important step was providing the board and executive leadership with information about succession planning programs in other nonhealthcare organizations that successfully maintained both organizational culture and profitability. Concretizing the types of skills that were seen as essential to effective leadership served to anchor the reality of the process.

As annual summaries of the succession planning program encompassed talent management and leadership development through the two-tiered program model, the benefits of the program were reinforced and the flow of the succession planning process was cascaded throughout all levels of leadership.

PREPARING AN ORGANIZATION FOR CHANGE

Implementing succession planning and leadership development may highlight the need (or create an opportunity) for strategic organizational restructuring. At BayCare, such a restructuring called for centralizing the executive leadership function of organization-wide departments in a way that ensured the CEO helmed the entire organization while managerial leaders still had a presence at each hospital site.

Broad change can be disruptive if the organization is not well prepared. Tuckman's (1965) model of how groups develop—forming, storming, norming, and performing—proved to be an excellent approach to preparing BayCare for such a monumental change. Centralizing the organization's executive leadership under a single individual was an enormous undertaking, but one that we felt was essential to offering excellent patient care.

- **Forming.** Bringing all members of the departments together to roll out the plans for centralization, drawing on the expert input from the team members who have been providing the service to the organization, and promoting a leader from within the ranks of the department all go a long way toward minimizing negative perceptions of the change.
- **Storming.** Any significant change brings with it the strong potential for resistance. Listening to questions, providing concrete answers, and helping individuals see the personal benefits will bring the organization through this phase of the change. This stage must not be glossed over or avoided, but rather embraced as part of the evolving process.
- **Norming.** As the processes for the integration of tasks, clarification of roles and responsibilities, and opportunities for a continual feedback loop unfold, the new processes become the norm.

- **Performing.** Continually seeking feedback, making modifications based on feedback, and acknowledging the benefits of the change reinforce the advantages both to the organization as a whole and to the individuals in the department.

PUBLIC VERSUS PRIVATE COMPANIES

The primary difference between a private organization and a publicly traded company is the accountability that a public company has to its shareholders. Public companies face tighter deadlines for measuring progress because they must report earnings on a quarterly basis and also face closer scrutiny of their expenditures.

Although succession planning will save an organization money in the long run, implementing a program may initially cause a small increase in the organization's operating expenses. Such expenses include the salaries of the Architect and any employees she may have, the cost of candidate assessments, and a small valuation of the time that succession planning participants spend on coaching and training (however, see our earlier discussion of salaried employees and the minimal impact succession planning has on productivity and job performance).

In the first few years, succession planning prepares candidates for internal promotion who generally are not yet ready to take on key leadership roles. While the succession planning program is maturing, the company still has to undertake costly searches for external candidates as leaders retire and their positions become available. The investment in a succession planning program will therefore not pay off for a few years; if a significant number of key leaders depart or retire during this period, it may appear as though the succession planning program is not having any effect beyond adding expenses that impact the bottom line. For public organizations that are focused on short-term earnings, these additional costs can prevent a board from supporting a succession planning program.

One strategy that public companies can use to overcome this obstacle is to create a full forecast of the long-term financial savings of a succession planning program, while simultaneously highlighting the potential costs involved in hiring external candidates. Painting a clearer picture of the organization's landscape five to ten years down the road may help public companies sway boards who are accustomed to thinking only three months ahead. A public company can also suggest implementing a strategy that keeps succession planning small at the outset, carefully selecting individuals who are likely to ascend to key leadership roles in the future. A smaller program could be handled directly by the Architect, who could add to her team only as needed for expansion to occur.

Case Study

As a healthcare system with 13 hospitals, BayCare faced the challenge of territorialism in the ranks of the medical records department at each hospital. Although some standardization had occurred as hospitals were integrated into the system, elements of uniqueness persisted among each department's staff, who felt that "this is how we do it here." The task of bringing together and forming a systemwide department required a leader with strong interpersonal skills and a commitment to excellence in a medical records arena. The implementation of the electronic medical record system at BayCare underscored the importance of a unified process.

The chosen leader for this process was selected from within the organization. She was a long-standing team member with a reputation for her commitment to quality service. She was also someone who was tolerant of the questions and challenges that accompany any significant change, and her capacity to relate to the situation was of great benefit. Her history of promotions

→

within the department had exposed her to many of the day-to-day nuances of medical records, and her ability to relate to questions such as "What is the impact on *my* job?" enhanced her credibility with the team members on the front line. As the change process unfolded, the clarification of roles, responsibilities, and reporting structure was as important to the norming stage as the standardizing elements of the medical record themselves were.

Taking into consideration the personal and structural impact of change, and seeking to address concerns openly and directly, is the foundation for an effective change process.

REFERENCES

Favaro, K., P. O. Karlsson, and G. L. Neilson. 2015. "The $112 Billion CEO Succession Problem." *Strategy + Business*. Published May 4. https://www.strategy-business.com/article/00327.

Tuckman, B. W. 1965. "Developmental Sequence in Small Groups." *Psychological Bulletin* 63 (6): 384–99.

PART II

Executing Succession Planning

CHAPTER 6

Referring Candidates to the Succession Planning Program

At this point, the why, when, who, what, and where of succession planning are in place (see exhibit 6.1). Your Visionary and Architect have teamed up, you've carefully crafted your succession planning program structure, and you've even gained the support of your company's board. Congratulations! The next step in succession planning is referring candidates to the program. From there, you can reassess, tweak, and modify the program structure as needed. You can also begin collecting feedback from the program on the candidates, which will be critical once you are ready to consider placing internal candidates in leadership roles.

As discussed in part I, we recommend making leadership development training mandatory for every employee in a leadership position. Not all of these leaders will join the succession planning program, so the referral process described in this chapter applies only to those who are referred. Also, a similar but distinct referral system may be used for employees who show leadership potential but do not currently hold a leadership role. A thorough discussion of these employees, whom we refer to as "Aspiring Leaders," appears in chapter 15.

Exhibit 6.1: Reviewing Why, When, Who, What, and Where

To create successful succession planning and leadership
development programs, you need only ask five critical questions:
Why? When? Who? What? Where?

Why
To develop a high-performing
organization driven by
personal leadership.

When
Start succession planning
immediately. A program takes
five to seven years to mature.

Who
A program must be led from the top
of the organization by two key
figures: the Visionary and the
Architect. Ultimately, it requires
commitment at all levels.

What
The program's structure and plan
for execution includes guidelines
for selection, training, coaching,
and feedback.

Where (it comes together)
Board commitment and support
are critical to implementing
succession planning and
leadership development.

A NOTE ON MAKING PROMISES YOU CAN—AND CAN'T—KEEP

You should always emphasize to participants in both succession planning and leadership development programs that (1) the goal is to help them become the best leaders possible in their current roles, and (2) the organization is making no promise of future promotion. It is particularly important that leaders selected for succession planning understand this concept before joining the program. Although their development will be individualized and is more likely to be geared toward a specific position, this is not a guarantee of ascendancy to a particular leadership role.

The Visionary, the Architect, and the Architect's team have a responsibility to avoid saying anything too soon about a participant's possible promotion. If you set the expectation that a succession planning participant will gain a certain title or position, you are taking an opportunity away from him because, if he focuses on a single path to advancement, he will close himself off to other chances for growth. Furthermore, a participant may consider herself a shoo-in for the next executive vacancy only to discover that two or three coworkers have also been preparing to be considered for the role.

This lack of guarantee may be frustrating for participants, and employees who don't see themselves moving up the ladder in the way they envisioned might even leave for other organizations. It is important to accept that the highest levels of leadership have a finite number of roles, and the timing of those roles' availability may not exactly fit a participant's personal career planning. However, in the process of developing each participant's competencies, the organization benefits significantly because that participant will be a more competent leader for as long as he or she remains an employee. If your leadership development program and company culture are strong, only a few people will depart for positions elsewhere. The tough reality is that if an employee is continually passed over for promotion, it is probably with good reason, and if the employee leaves, you likely will not be losing one of your company's more valuable assets.

REFERRING CANDIDATES

We discussed some alternatives for referring candidates to the succession planning program in chapter 4. At the outset of our succession planning program, we solicited referrals for the program directly from our level A executives. As explained earlier, we included executives at levels A, B, and C in succession planning, but only to replace positions at levels A and B. Even so, we found that the level A leaders didn't have a day-to-day working knowledge of the competencies of the people outside of their specific area. As a result, we sought input from human resources to identify high-potential candidates and then approached the leaders to whom these individuals reported to confirm the appropriateness of their referral to succession planning. By the third and fourth years, most members of our leadership team knew about the program and were reaching out to the Architect to recommend their direct reports for succession planning. The method of soliciting referrals from the top executive layer naturally progressed to a more effective system in which the referral now comes from the individual's manager.

> Referrals should always go through an individual's direct manager because that manager will, in all likelihood, end up being the candidate's coach. Not only does the candidate commit to the program, but the manager commits to facilitating the candidate's success as well. The manager sees the candidate day in, day out and has the greatest opportunity to make an impact through both formal and informal coaching.
>
> —Kathie

As our program expanded to include more levels of leadership, we officially transitioned to the method of directly soliciting our management team to refer their direct reports to succession planning. We use this same referral process for the Aspiring Leader track of leadership development, which is for employees who are not currently in leadership roles and is thus elective instead of compulsory (remember, all current leaders are already receiving leadership development). We suggest using the management-led referral model because this format not only helps obtain the most viable candidates but also makes it an honor to be selected and invited into the program.

A succession planning candidate not only must perform well on assessments but also must display the qualities of strong leadership daily at work. A candidate's direct boss is the best person to notice and report this kind of behavior. The referral process also acts as a filter to keep program numbers lower than they would be under a self-referral process.

Once succession planning catches on, you may have to contend with eager employees stopping you in the hallway and asking to be a part of your program. Acknowledge their excitement and ask them to speak with their boss about making the necessary referral. In rare circumstances, the Architect or Visionary might notice a stellar individual and approach this employee's manager directly for a referral. In all cases, however, the manager is an integral part of a candidate's selection for succession planning.

> Once our succession planning program began expanding, I quickly realized that executive leaders, including myself, were not the best people to refer candidates to the program. We didn't have adequate firsthand knowledge of and experience with candidates. Fortunately, we were able to rely on our managers in this regard.
>
> —Steve

CHAPTER 7

Assessing Candidates

ONCE A CANDIDATE has been accepted into the succession planning program, he or she will take the full assessment battery that the Architect has selected. As discussed in chapter 4, we recommend administering the assessments only after the candidate has been accepted into the program rather than as a determining factor for program admittance. When introducing the succession planning program to the organization, it is helpful to distinguish between the assessment process for the program and employees' annual performance appraisals. Although the ongoing performance of a succession planning participant will be gradually integrated into the perception of his or her readiness for promotion, the initial assessment battery encompasses competencies that are different from those used to measure annual performance. Likewise, candidates need to be confident that the results of the assessment battery will not negatively affect their annual performance reviews.

In chapter 3, we discussed the qualifications the Architect needs to be able to select and administer these assessments. As the succession planning program expands, the Architect will find it helpful if members of her team are also certified in administering and interpreting the assessments. More information about the Architect's team is provided in chapter 16.

> It's vital that the Architect have a working knowledge of which assessments are most appropriate for candidates in a succession planning program. That will differ for each organization.
>
> —Kathie

ASSESSMENT SKILL SETS AND COMPETENCIES

Once selected by the Architect, the assessment battery is used to create a picture of a candidate's current competencies and to get a sense of his or her strengths and growth opportunities. This information will be used to tailor an executive development plan (EDP), which may include specialized training or assignments to foster growth in specific areas. Typically, the assessment battery is used to determine the following four skill sets:

1. **Intrapersonal.** Intrapersonal skills relate to one's understanding of oneself. To lead others, a leader must possess both self-awareness and self-confidence, which can be combined in the concept of "self-trust." If you don't trust yourself, it is extremely difficult for other people to find you trustworthy, especially when you are in a leadership position. An intrapersonal assessment also establishes an individual's baseline—who the individual is at his or her very core. As a leader, every candidate will face challenges and difficulties, and in moments of intense stress, we all revert to our baseline behavioral patterns. Knowing how a candidate *will* act in a given situation, not how the candidate thinks he or she *should* act, is what's important.

2. **Interpersonal.** Interpersonal skills refer to how an individual relates to and interacts with people. This includes the ability to communicate well with others—for example, a leader's ability to clearly articulate what she

expects from her direct reports. Listening skills are also important, because leaders need to be capable of open dialogue with their employees. Leaders additionally need to be able to listen to criticism and feedback from their superiors and apply that feedback in a constructive way. Interpersonal skills also relate to the way a leader works with others, such as collaborating with other departments to put together a presentation for the CEO or the company's board.

3. **Emotional intelligence.** The third component of the assessment battery is emotional intelligence, which, in a sense, synthesizes both intrapersonal and interpersonal skills. Emotional intelligence is a leader's ability to identify, understand, and make decisions based on someone's feelings or emotional state—both the leader's own feelings and those of his or her employees. Individuals who possess high emotional intelligence are able to manage their own feelings effectively, display sensitivity to the needs of others, and understand somebody else's mood. Emotional intelligence fosters compassionate communication, reduces conflict, and supports a positive work environment.

4. **360-degree for "hard" skills.** A 360-degree feedback assessment covers the full competencies in which candidates for succession planning will need to demonstrate skills. Data are collected from one's self, boss, direct reports, peers, and others regarding various leadership competencies. By collecting data on an individual from multiple sources for the same set of criteria, you obtain a clear picture of that individual's performance as a leader across all strata of his or her relationships. The 360-degree assessment emphasizes hard skills such as strategic planning, visionary thinking, and forecasting but also includes some relational competencies, or "soft" skills.

ROUNDING OUT THE LEADERSHIP PROFILE

In addition to the assessment battery, candidates should submit their resume as part of their leadership profile. The Architect or a member of her team will also need to conduct a structured interview with the candidate. (As described in chapter 21, we recommend that the emotional intelligence assessment take place within this structured interview framework, although a wide variety of emotional intelligence tests are available.) The structured interview allows the Architect's team to understand the individual's goals and personality and to answer any questions that the candidate may have. This interview is also an opportunity to review the expectations of the succession planning program very clearly, to make certain the candidate thoroughly understands the process and what will be required.

CHAPTER 8

Placing Candidates in Succession Planning

ONCE A CANDIDATE has completed the assessment battery, he or she is provided with extensive feedback. Candidates are asked to take several weeks to review this feedback and then select three or four competency areas where they would like to grow and expand their skills. Although the Architect or a member of her team will also have reviewed the reports and identified areas for development, the final decision rests with the candidate. From here, the candidate's executive development plan (EDP) is created, and the candidate becomes a participant in succession planning.

The EDP guides the participant toward achieving goals and improving specific competencies. All the elements of succession planning, as well as the leadership development curriculum the individual is required to participate in, are included in the EDP. Additionally, every EDP should contain the goal of developing others, because this supports the cascading nature of succession planning in the organization.

Initially, the Architect is responsible for writing the EDP for every candidate entering the succession planning program. As the program expands, however, the Architect should acquire a team. We recommend that team members be certified as executive coaches; with this training, they not only will become more skilled as coaches but will also learn to write EDPs so that the Architect is not solely responsible for this work.

Writing an EDP requires the capacity to interpret and integrate findings from a variety of sources. You must look at what the participant knows about herself, how that plays into her interactions with others, and what implications it has for her as a leader, including areas where she may need to engage more and micromanage less.

Structurally, a succession planning participant's EDP will include three primary elements: training, coaching, and supplemental resources. While training and coaching are also primary elements of the leadership development program that supports succession planning, supplemental resources are typically reserved for participants in succession planning because individuals in the talent pipeline are early in their careers and have less need for highly individualized programming; EDPs, on the other hand, are highly individualized. Although certain leadership competencies may be required of all leaders in the organization, the approach to development is unique to each participant.

TRAINING

Before presenting the succession planning program to the board, the Architect and Visionary will have mapped out the specific leadership competencies that participants are expected to demonstrate. Some of these competencies will be developed through leadership training, which we recommend for all leaders in the organization, not just those in succession planning. At the outset, creating one standard leadership training module for all leaders is easiest; once the program has expanded, the training can be modified to coordinate with differentiated leadership tracks. This standardized leadership training is only one part of a succession planning participant's EDP, other aspects of which will address competencies and areas for growth that are specific to the individual.

In general, an EDP's training recommendations should develop core cultural competencies that all leaders in the organizations need to possess, as well as any other skills specific to an individual leader. Training and certifications may be created based on the particular values of your company or modeled on the coursework of organizations such as Development Dimensions International, the Franklin Covey Institute, and the Center for Leadership Studies. For example, the EDP for an individual who has growth opportunities around "driving execution" might contain a strategy to attend a Covey "5 Choices" workshop.

The Visionary and Architect must carefully consider the amount of time, effort, and resources that leadership training will require of the participant, his or her coach, the Architect's team, and the organization overall. If certification is required for all leaders at a certain level, then you should clearly lay out the timeline for obtaining the certification, as well as the repercussions for not being certified within the designated time frame.

At BayCare, we required an internal leadership certification for all leaders at levels A–D (see exhibit 4.1). Under this system, an individual is expected to complete the core classes within one year of hire or promotion. If the leader chooses to take elective classes on change management, conflict, and mediation, she has an additional year to complete the certification process, as well as a capstone course that measures competency in the skills taught in the classes. We discuss how we restructured and improved our leadership certification in detail in chapter 12.

You should also consider who will teach the leadership courses and how often they will be offered. If your company opts to keep leadership training in-house, then this responsibility will fall on the Architect, and to her team if she has one. Although you can send participants to external leadership training or hire a consulting company to provide courses and workshops, we strongly recommend that the Architect and her team conduct in-house training, for several reasons.

First, using external resources or a consulting company will quickly and significantly increase the program's costs, which may present additional difficulties in gaining the support of your board. Second, having the Architect and her support team create in-house training ensures that the content is in step with your organization's cultural competencies and values. Finally, in-house training allows your organization to control the language and presentation of material, encouraging participants to develop a common vocabulary when speaking about leadership. This sense of "speaking the same language" promotes enhanced communication among leaders in the company.

COACHING

Every EDP in our organization assigns a coach. The coaching component of the succession planning program, and of leadership development overall, allows participants the opportunity to synthesize and use the skills and lessons learned in their leadership training and to have the guidance of a coach when working on strategies outlined in their development plans. Coaching also gives employees the opportunity to work through situations that arise on the job in real time. Coaches work closely with succession plannng participants to provide opportunities for expanded responsibilities that will help them acquire or enhance competencies as outlined in their EDP. Following a structured approach, the coach reinforces the participant's recognition of strengths and uses this recognition as a platform for further development. The participant's career aspirations are discussed during coaching sessions so that the coach has a clear understanding of what type of experiences and training would be most beneficial.

The coach also provides feedback on the participant's progress, helps to course-correct strategies as circumstances change, and explores creative solutions to obstacles and barriers that arise. Through coaching, participants refine their thinking and learn to view the future as a place of possibility. Setting and achieving goals promotes self-confidence and self-esteem, and development of these qualities builds and maintains the culture of the entire organization.

Who acts as coach? The most desirable and sustainable model is to have participants coached by the person to whom they directly report, or by a key leadership executive whose areas of expertise the participant desires to be exposed to in order to acquire similar competencies. Daily interaction and observation of participants by their boss provides the most substantial venue for development to be monitored and guided.

Our own emphasis on coaching began with the organization-wide communication of the expectation that leaders would focus on the development of their direct reports. This communication was initiated in the management orientation process—a multiday orientation on leadership fundamentals that is required of all newly hired or promoted leaders. Additionally, a class in our leadership training was devoted to a framework for coaching that provided strategies and tools for carrying out this expectation. Thus, by the time individuals entered the succession planning program, the importance of coaching—both for themselves and for their direct reports—had been deeply ingrained into their understanding of leadership roles in the organization's culture.

In larger organizations, opportunities exist for the Architect and her team to provide additional coaching, particularly when a participant requires more targeted competency development. The adjunct coaching is coordinated closely with the participant's central coach, with the overarching goal of helping the participant better lead his team.

Coaching also reinforces the coach's own leadership development. This model is based on the principle that one of the best ways to learn is by teaching others. When a coach helps a participant apply leadership principles and philosophy, she in turn strengthens her own connection to and understanding of those same principles. Knowing that she is leading by example as a manager, she also has a high degree of accountability for living the values of leadership every day at work. Additionally, the coach and the participant are likely to be in the same department and therefore share a common vocabulary when it comes to understanding specific issues that arise on the job.

Even with a foundation established by management orientation and leadership training programs, some leaders still find that coaching poses considerable challenges. In such situations, the Architect and her team can practice a process of "coaching the coaches," helping leaders lead more effectively. We want leaders to use their leadership skills in helping, directing, and mentoring others. (We further discuss creating a team of coaches in chapter 17.)

When you first launch a succession planning program, all participants will likely be higher-level executives. As such, the one-on-one coaching model is most effective. The opportunity to have private sessions with a coach gives program participants, who may be preparing to take on significant leadership roles in the company within a few years, the chance to improve specific competencies that they may need to accelerate their career tracks. Through individualized EDPs, participants work on goals established to address identified competency gaps. The coaching process is one of dual responsibility: The leader is expected to be accountable for seeking out coaching for his own development, and the coach is expected to provide opportunities for development through expanded roles, stretch assignments, or specific training options.

COACHING THE CEO

For the Visionary, who is likely the CEO, the model of being coached by one's direct manager is not effective—he is at the top of the organization. Yet, the Visionary may still benefit from coaching, and it's here that the Board Advocate or other board members may step in to offer advisory assistance. The organization may also hire an external coach for the Visionary or have him work with consultants who can provide guidance.

PROVIDING SUPPLEMENTAL RESOURCES

Occasionally, succession planning participants have specific skills or competencies designated as growth areas that fall outside the boundaries of the general leadership curriculum. These growth areas may represent a gap in individual development, or they may be areas that are not required for the participant's current role but may be a part of a future role in the organization. For example, an individual might be a visionary thinker but lack financial acumen, which could impact strategy development for pursuing his vision. The Architect and the individual's coach can work together to create specialized assignments designed to improve his financial acumen, a mentor around finance might be recommended, or he might be referred to additional training or external workshops.

Mentorship as an adjunct to coaching can help address a participant's specific needs for leadership development. In some instances, a coach may not have the skills to help the participant grow in a particular area—for example, if the participant is preparing to transition to another department in the company. In addition to a coach, the participant might also be assigned a mentor who has the skills and knowledge to help the participant grow in a specific area or competency. The need for a mentor might also arise if the individual and her direct superior have different approaches to development and a mentor can most appropriately fill in the gaps.

Occasionally, a participant may struggle with developing his leadership competencies. This tends to show up in coaching sessions, where processing emotions and receiving feedback can create sensitive circumstances. A participant may be dealing with deep-seated issues of confidence and self-trust that need to be addressed before he can make significant progress in developing new skills and competencies. You should make it clear to all coaches that they can call on the Architect and her team if a participant is having significant difficulty with the program. The Architect may suggest that the participant work with one of her certified coaches to better understand the issues at hand.

On rare occasions, an Architect with the appropriate credentials in psychology may be able to recommend supportive therapy. Although an organization cannot mandate that a succession planning participant attend therapy, we have found that when we show a commitment to individuals by providing such supplemental resources, they generally reciprocate with a commitment to follow through with the support or additional training they need. The scenario in which a participant is recommended for therapy is not common; in the more than ten years that our succession planning program has existed, there have been only two instances of such referrals.

PART III

Succession Planning in Action

CHAPTER 9

Replacing a Key Leader

ON SECURING THE board's approval, there is plenty of work to be done. The Architect must now put into action the plan she has carefully laid out, while the Visionary must communicate the purpose and benefits of the succession planning program to the entire organization. Succession planning typically unfolds from the top down, and the Board Advocate will first want to ensure that a plan for the CEO is put into place.

As the program picks up steam, the Architect should provide regular progress reports to the board. Communicating with the board on a quarterly basis is a good rule of thumb, and the Board Advocate should be willing to liaise with the Visionary, Architect, and board as needed. Inviting board members to participate in any open leadership training or education being provided to the organization can also be beneficial, because it allows them to experience leadership development in action.

Let's fast-forward five years. Assume that you have successfully crafted and implemented your succession planning program for the top levels of executive leadership in your organization. Succession planning participants are receiving coaching and training on an ongoing basis, and they are developing specific competencies that may help them take on new roles in the company. Suppose that around this time (and hopefully not before), a key leader of the company announces her impending retirement. The Visionary and the Architect decide that the program has matured enough to evaluate internal candidates and to identify one as her potential replacement. You are now ready to put your succession planning program to the ultimate test.

REVISITING A DEPARTING LEADER'S ROLE

Replacing a key leader requires the same clarity and focus necessary for achieving any other business goal: You must know exactly what you are aiming at before you can hit the target. When a key leader announces her departure, the first step is to become crystal clear about that leader's role in the company. You are not merely searching for a candidate who is like the previous executive; you are seeking a candidate who meets the precise requirements for the position the executive is vacating. The departing leader herself may be vital to this process, because her perceptions about what her role's key competencies are can be used to establish a baseline. Even though an organization may not always be looking for a candidate who is like the previous executive in terms of skill sets, ultimately the incoming employee should be like-minded with respect to the organization's values and its vision of where the company is headed.

This is when the vocabulary and structure of leadership development step in. Under the umbrella of leadership development, you have already created and defined specific competencies that are valuable to leaders in your organization, and your succession planning participants have been improving these skills for half a decade. The Visionary and Architect should together decide which of these competencies are most vital for the position being vacated and, from there, create an articulate description of what qualifications the next candidate needs to fill the role.

This description should be created based on the role itself, not the specific duties, competencies, or behaviors of the individual leaving the role. The departing leader may have had responsibilities that are no longer appropriate based on the organization's current structure; likewise, an incoming leader may need additional skills because of organizational restructuring or shifts in the industry. A departure in key leadership is always an opportunity to examine a role with fresh eyes and to determine what is most important in that role for the company *now*.

As you go through this examination process, you might recognize that you want to shift a position's requirements because your company's internal structure has changed. Management reorganization might mean that a position reports somewhere new, that it has suddenly risen from level C to level B, or even that it is no longer needed.

You might also revise a role's description because the market conditions surrounding your business have changed. You might determine that the next executive will focus on emerging market trends rather than maintain the status quo of the past ten years. A shift in market trends will likely require the next candidate to possess new or different skill sets, such as being tech savvy or emphasizing cost savings instead of fee generation. Taking the time to thoroughly evaluate the skills that the position will require in the next few years is critical as you identify the candidate who is the best fit for the organization. The Visionary plays a key role in this process, because he is responsible for considering the future and anticipating what the company will look like down the line.

A perfect example of revising a role's qualifications could happen in healthcare. We anticipate a major shift in the healthcare market—namely, a transition from volume-based reimbursement of services to a payment system that rewards value, which is calculated as quality of service divided by cost. Under one value-based payment model, a healthcare organization would receive a lump sum from Medicare or an insurance company to restore and maintain a patient's

> Healthcare is facing significant shifts in its business model right now. As a result, some of our leadership roles are being retooled to better prepare organizations for the future.
> —Steve

health. At the end of the year, the provider would get to keep any amount not spent on that patient, and it would have to absorb any overexpenditure. In other words, we anticipate a 180-degree shift in the way providers think about care delivery and their organization's bottom line.

Let's assume your organization is aware that a longtime level B executive is planning to retire before age 67. If a strong succession planning program is in place, your organization would start a conversation with him well in advance of his retirement. It would work with the executive to find mutually agreeable terms for the timing of the departure and appropriate accommodations for a transition. Ideally, the person who takes his position would start six months before the executive departs to allow some overlap. But the amount of time is variable and depends on the departing executive, the new candidate, and the role she is taking over.

Once you have begun this conversation with the retiring executive, you should review his position and determine which competencies are most important for the next candidate in the role. You should consider what the current leader's focus was, the main value he brought to the organization, and the specific skills that made him successful. Keeping this information in mind, and anticipating the forecasted skill requirements for the next ten years, map the desired skills of the current role and add any additional competencies required to meet expected future challenges.

You may know from the start of this process that you need an individual who brings a different mind-set to the table to adapt to the evolving goals of the organization. In such a scenario, you will undoubtedly find that the requirements for an incoming executive look quite different from the skill sets of the retiring executive.

Crafting a clear role description before replacing someone also allows you to hold candidates to a fixed, measurable standard. Rather than being compared to one another ("I think John is better than Cindy, but not as good as Doreen"), candidates are measured against the rubric of what the position requires. If a candidate does not meet this objective standard, then you know that the search to fill the position is not yet over. Although demanding, the rubric test ensures that you hire someone who can truly excel in the role and not settle for someone who is merely good enough to get the job done.

Occasionally, you may have a role requirement that affects all new leaders organization-wide. For instance, BayCare decided to require all level A–D leaders to complete leadership training and develop the competency of coaching and developing others. These skills are so important to us that any new employees hired into a leadership position moved directly from management orientation to leadership development. These qualities were built right into their job descriptions, as well as the company's DNA.

The Visionary, Architect, and Board Advocate may all be involved in crafting the key leader job description. For example, if the role being examined is the CEO, then the Visionary, as the current individual in that role, will have significant input as to the position's requirements. The Board Advocate may also have an opinion about what the board needs from an incoming top-level executive. Input from the Visionary and the Board Advocate may also be applicable to other roles, such as chief operating officer or chief financial officer (CFO). For leadership positions outside the top tier of executives, the Board Advocate is less likely to have direct input regarding the job description. The Visionary may still be involved to some extent, particularly if the description is being revised based on a new direction in which the Visionary is leading the company. The Architect is always involved in this process because she and her team facilitate every leadership transition and because her background gives her expertise in understanding the skills required for specific roles. Other individuals who may be involved, depending on the role, include the team member who currently occupies that role and her direct manager. Who exactly is involved will vary from position to position and, as mentioned, will depend on whether the role is being revised to incorporate new strategic shifts in the organization.

REPLACING THE CEO

The CEO—who, for the purposes of this book, is also typically the Visionary—is the most important leader whose role an organization needs to fill. You have likely heard horror stories about companies whose CEOs departed under dramatic, tragic, or scandalous circumstances. Such exits create significant instability in the company and can do lasting damage to both an organization's culture and its bottom line.

> Succession planning became a real issue for our board when we started talking about who would replace Steve, our CEO, after his retirement.
>
> —Larry

Let's examine three common ways the CEO transition can occur. You will see not only how succession planning can improve each scenario but also how it can create a CEO transition that is as stable and smooth as possible.

The first two scenarios describe what might happen in the event of a CEO's departure when a strong and active succession planning program is not in place:

I. **The crisis.** In a crisis, the CEO departs unexpectedly. This most frequently occurs because of sudden illness or death. More rarely, the CEO decides to leave the organization without any warning.

In an unplanned departure, the company's board plays a critical role by stepping in to fill the position. Board members face a host of problems when the CEO position is vacated unexpectedly and no succession planning program is in place. Specifically, the board is under extreme pressure to find a replacement quickly, which may mean there is not enough time to appropriately vet candidates or to get a clear picture of the role's requirements. Unless the CEO died or experienced a sudden health crisis, prospective candidates might have concerns about the CEO's departure, particularly if it happened under mysterious circumstances, and the organization might have trouble attracting top talent for the position. Finally, the disarray could cause company morale to plummet if employees believe the company's leaders don't have a clear plan in place.

2. **Board-driven change.** Board-driven change arises when the organization's board determines that the current CEO is no longer a good fit for the position and decides to seek a new candidate for the role. Depending on the circumstances, the board may have some leeway in finding a replacement, but occasionally they may ask the CEO to step down immediately.

   A number of the challenges presented by a board-driven CEO change are similar to those in the crisis scenario: The organization is thrown into tumult, the board has to make hasty decisions, and morale may significantly decline. Additionally, board-driven change can create rifts within the board itself, as all board members rarely agree that a CEO should be replaced. This conflict can lead to infighting and strife at a moment when the board needs to present a strong, unified front to the organization.

In the two scenarios just described, it's clear that a lack of planning combined with unexpected circumstances can lead to organizational chaos. But consider what would change if the organization has a succession plan in place. Although the sudden nature of the crisis scenario cannot be avoided, a candidate would likely be ready (or nearly ready) to step into the CEO role. The board could provide additional support to that individual as needed, but she would already understand where the company was going and what the organization required. Under the board-driven change scenario, at least one individual would be ready to step into the role whether the CEO departed swiftly or agreed to leave a few months down the road. In the latter case, a candidate could be selected from the succession planning program and ample resources spent preparing him to replace the CEO. Although both scenarios would still be rocky, succession planning could significantly improve the transitions.

Let's turn now to a third scenario, which is the one every organization hopes for: a well-planned transition to the new CEO.

3. **The planned succession.** In the planned-succession scenario, the organization creates a clear timeline for transitioning from one CEO to the next. This approach includes determining who will replace the CEO and adequately preparing that individual to take over the role before the transition happens. Because the CEO is also likely the Visionary, he should feel comfortable talking about his own replacement and providing input on how the transition will happen. The members of the board will also play a key role here, as they will be invested in setting up a transition that works well not only for the individuals involved but also for the organization itself. With ample time and resources, the board may be able to dedicate a committee to planning for the succession of the CEO, and of course, the Architect will facilitate every step of the process. If a succession planning program has matured by the time a CEO transition occurs, an internal candidate will likely be found to assume the role. If so, the current and future CEOs can work together to ensure that the future CEO is prepared to take over the role.

    Although a planned succession may not always be possible, it is certainly the preferred situation for transitioning the role of CEO. Regardless of how the CEO departs, a succession planning program makes the possibility of a smooth transition much more likely.

WHEN IS AN EXTERNAL SEARCH APPROPRIATE?

A strong succession planning program supported by a strong leadership development program can dramatically increase the number of candidates your company promotes from within. However, we want to make it clear that the company's goal should never be to promote exclusively from its own pool of individuals. No organization can thrive long-term on an internal-promotion-only policy because there is too much commonality of mind-set. Even companies with the strongest culture and values need some outside perspectives to offer new opinions, challenge them to grow, and push the boundaries of change. We set the goal of flipping our organization from a 20-to-80 ratio of hiring internal versus external candidates to an 80-to-20 ratio.

In certain circumstances when an executive retires, an external search will likely produce the best candidates for the job because skills are needed that your organization, and therefore your leaders, simply have not been honing for the past five to ten years. At times, strategic initiatives will require you to bring someone with a different viewpoint into the fold.

You still want to be sure that an external candidate will fit in well with the company's culture. You want to be confident that anybody you hire has a mind-set consistent with your organization's values. In our case, for example, all leaders need to be willing to coach and develop their direct reports. This is a vital part of our company's mind-set, and a candidate who brings a fresh perspective to the table but is unwilling to embrace our value system will ultimately not be the right fit.

You might also consider hiring an external candidate to diversify the organization's leadership. Many companies succeed at increasing the number of internal candidates who are promoted but fail to make significant gains in including women and individuals from racially and ethnically diverse backgrounds. If diversity is an area of growth for your organization, you will need to make a conscious effort to move away from the status quo of your current leadership team. Long-term succession planning will foster greater diversity by helping individuals rise from all levels in the company, as opposed to merely boosting those who are already in leadership roles into key leadership positions.

Some roles in an organization, such as the CFO, are singular. A CFO needs a broad base of knowledge and experience in addition to expert financial acumen. An organization whose field is narrowly focused may find an internal candidate who is suitable for the position fairly quickly, but a large organization with many moving parts may not initially have an internal candidate who is sufficiently cross-trained to replace a CFO. As the larger organization's succession planning program matures, however, the time invested in cross-training level B leaders in the finance department will more likely produce a viable candidate.

Fostering a mind-set of internal promotion should never mean that a position is filled by a candidate just because she already works for the company. Your job is to create the strongest leadership team possible for your organization, not to promote from within regardless of skill level or qualifications. A strong succession planning program supported by an equally strong leadership development program will create internal candidates who are the best fit for taking on key leadership roles.

MOVING UP THE LADDER—LATERALLY

"Moving up the corporate ladder" is not a steady, linear journey; the path is frequently circuitous. Sometimes an individual will move into a key leadership role only after holding a number of different positions. Within the framework of a succession planning program, you may move participants *laterally* in the short term to prepare them to make *ladder* moves later on. In other words, an individual might be cross-promoted, shifting within a department or even changing departments altogether, without gaining a higher title or bigger office. The lateral move helps her gain more breadth of experience, and then, when a ladder move with a new title and more responsibility becomes available, she has the credentials to be considered for that position.

Lateral versus ladder moves are generally discussed as part of the coaching process. It is a time to help the participant understand the benefits of looking laterally within the organization to broaden his experience base and be a more desirable candidate when a ladder promotion becomes available. The coach and participant can work on this process together, but it is the participant's responsibility to be on the lookout for opportunities throughout the organization and take the initiative to explore them. When you approach the process from this perspective, participants usually display little resistance and embrace the opportunity to learn new skills.

By way of example, imagine that you have a lateral-to-ladder move in your organization. You have an employee who occupies a position within a narrow reporting structure, with a single function that offers no upward mobility. To expand his potential span of exposure and support his leadership and skill development, this employee's role is shifted so that instead of reporting to a level A leader, he now reports to a level B executive. Although it may not seem like a promotion, the shift could expand his role considerably. It would allow him to gain significant experience in other areas and develop skills that may be critical for a ladder promotion in the next few years. Although the short-term move is not up the ladder, the long-term future of this employee could be very bright.

CHAPTER 10

Internal Versus External Candidates

ONCE YOU HAVE clarified the specific role requirements for the position you are filling, you can return to the Architect for her expertise. During the past five to ten years, she has been gathering data, observing and working with coaches, leading workshops and training sessions, and managing whatever issues arise in the succession planning program. The question you now pose to the Architect is: Does our organization have any internal candidates who could fill this role?

DRAFTING THE SHORT LIST

To answer your question, the Architect turns to the data she has collected. In general, succession planning participants who are one to two levels below the position being filled are under consideration as candidates. It is unlikely that a level D candidate would be skyrocketed to a level A position; the candidate's competencies and experience for the role simply aren't yet developed. However, a level B or even a high-achieving level C candidate could be considered for the role. Part of creating a short list involves looking at potential candidates' annual performance appraisals, which emphasize the organization's cultural beliefs. Reviewing their performance appraisals gives the Architect insight as to how the candidates are reinforcing the organization's values and quality culture on a daily basis.

After the Architect identifies possible candidates for consideration, she then meets directly with the candidates' coaches. This allows her to obtain more information about the day-to-day experience of working with each candidate, to determine whether the candidate is open or resistant to coaching, and to ascertain the candidate's specific leadership competencies—all information that will supplement the data from the candidate's annual performance appraisal. The coaches help the Architect identify candidates' skills, capabilities, and areas for growth. The Architect may also consult her own team members if they facilitated a workshop or leadership training with the candidates.

When the fact-finding mission is complete, the Architect prepares a short list of candidates to be considered for filling the vacant position. This selection process is ultimately driven by the competencies required and the role description created for the vacant position, as described in chapter 9. Once the competencies have been mapped out, they become the standard against which every candidate's skill set is measured.

After creating the short list, the Architect and her team step back and let human resources take over, inviting candidates to interview for the position and facilitating the interviews. The interview process for a level A candidate typically consists of a series of interviews involving human resources, the other level A leaders, a couple board members, and four or five direct reports. The process shifts as you get to lower levels of the organization; the CEO would not, for example, generally be involved in interviewing candidates for a level C position.

If a clear internal candidate for the position emerges from the interview process, he is offered the new job and the process is complete. In situations where a suitable internal candidate is not found—usually because all candidates need to further develop their competencies—the internal search concludes and an external candidate search begins.

Advances in technology now offer streamlined solutions for tracking candidates and creating short lists of viable candidates as positions become available. (See chapter 12 for more information.)

AVOIDING HEAD-TO-HEAD COMPETITION

We consider it extremely important not to pit internal and external candidates directly against one another. In fact, once our succession planning program had achieved a certain depth, we established a company policy that a review of internal candidates would automatically happen first when a level A or level B position became available. Only if no viable candidates surfaced from an internal review would we then post the position externally. This policy reinforced the message that we were deeply committed to succession planning and that we gave our internal candidates the chance to succeed whenever possible.

Some organizations regularly consider internal and external candidates together in the same recruitment process. This may work out to be advantageous for the internal candidates, but when it doesn't, internal candidates face a significant career challenge. This kind of direct competition can foster bitterness and resentment, particularly if the internal candidate remains with the organization after not being selected for promotion. Additionally, combining internal and external candidates in the same pool can prevent external candidates from building strong working relationships—for example, with members of the organization's board who preferred an internal candidate for the position.

By evaluating internal candidates first, the board clearly sees whether any existing employees have the abilities necessary to fill a vacant role. If not, employees and board members alike can move on, and the external search can take place with less friction. Part of the value of succession planning is its approach to leadership change, which meaningfully measures skills and competencies, promotes camaraderie, and avoids unnecessary conflict in the organization.

CHAPTER 11

Timing the Replacement of a Leader

THE PROCESS OF replacing a leader takes time, and the higher the leadership role, the longer it takes. Although in many organizations the key leaders (levels A and B for our purposes) are required to provide only 30 days' notice before leaving, in practice we recommend discussing retirement with all key leaders well in advance of their anticipated departure. Most people who care about their legacy are comfortable with these conversations, and the succession planning culture helps normalize this process.

For planned departures, ongoing discussion allows plenty of time for the Architect to create a short list of internal candidates and for human resources to review and interview them (and still conduct an external search, if necessary). If an internal candidate is selected to fill the position, the entire process takes approximately three months. A search for an external candidate, on the other hand, might take nine months or more. An external candidate search includes all of the elements of an internal search plus hiring a consultant, culling a list of approximately 50 candidates, interviewing the top 8, picking the top 3 for a second round of interviews, and sometimes repeating the entire process if no viable candidate emerges. The scheduling alone is an enormous undertaking and can create significant delays.

One benefit of promoting an internal candidate, especially one who is selected well in advance, is that she has the opportunity to shadow or be mentored by the leader she is replacing. This allows her to experience the rhythm, pace, and particulars of the new position before bearing full responsibility for the role. This kind of opportunity is generally not available to external hires, whose first day on the job may not be until after the previous leader has departed. Even if there is some overlap between the retiring executive and the new external hire, financial considerations may limit the amount of time an external candidate can spend with her predecessor.

Additionally, internal candidates can concentrate on any specific competencies they may need to develop before assuming a new position in the organization. When you use the rubric of a role's description as a quality standard, as opposed to comparing candidates with one another, you may find that a candidate is a great fit for the job but needs focused training in one or two specific skills to tackle the position's full responsibilities with confidence. Once identified for the position, an internal candidate might spend three to six months honing those skills before fully taking on the role, potentially supported by coaching from the departing leader herself. In contrast, an external hire may not start until after the previous leader has left, so any skill set development will happen only after he assumes his new position.

When the leader being replaced is the CEO or another head executive, some additional considerations may affect the timing of the transition. It is even more pivotal that your current CEO's departure is discussed well in advance of any transition; two or more years is ideal. Having some measure of flexibility around a CEO's departure is also beneficial, because the timing of the handoff depends on both external and internal factors, such as the following in healthcare:

- **Product life cycle.** Healthcare's current emphasis on providing more services to obtain greater revenue is changing, albeit slowly, to a focus on keeping people healthy to achieve greater savings. This change from volume to value represents the end of one product life cycle and the beginning of another. Any major executive transition during this time should take the product life cycle into account.

- **Government regulations.** A perfect example of government regulation is the Affordable Care Act (ACA), which has had major consequences for healthcare. Steve's own transition out of the CEO role and into retirement was timed around implementation of the ACA, to ensure his organization was stable during this time of industry upheaval.
- **Repositioning in the organization.** An organization might move in a new direction because of an industry-wide shift or developments in technology. In healthcare, an industry shift could be placing greater emphasis on preventive services, while a technological development could be a company's pivot to focus on telehealth options for patients.

> Whenever possible, we like to see current team members fill available leadership positions. They understand our mission and our values in a way that external candidates often don't.
>
> —Steve

PART IV

Scaling and Refining Succession Planning and Leadership Development

CHAPTER 12

Pivots, U-Turns, and Tune-Ups

WE WILL BE the first to tell you that the process of implementing succession planning and leadership development programs involves a significant amount of trial and error. The process must be dynamic and ever-changing to meet the evolving needs of the organization, and its leaders must therefore be flexible, adaptable, and humble. We can point to several examples of shifts and improvements we made at BayCare over the past decade, as well as advances our successors are moving toward in the next few years.

One of the most significant examples in our organization is covered thoroughly later in this chapter. In brief, we began with a leadership training program that was fundamentally based in an educational framework, but we realized we wanted to expand the experiential aspect of the classes while respecting the time that leaders had for professional development. We also shifted the emphasis of the leadership certification so that it established a firm foundation for our company's quality culture.

Chapter 6 alludes to a lesson we learned early on in succession planning, when we asked only a small core of level A leaders to refer candidates to the program. We quickly realized that these leaders did not have a sufficiently broad knowledge of leadership at deeper levels in the organization and were therefore not able to refer candidates with confidence. We course-corrected that process, initially by soliciting our head of human resources for referrals. This system eventually evolved into the referral system we recommend in this book, whereby candidates are referred by their direct superior. This maturation created a program that now has a much broader awareness of individuals and their abilities.

Moving forward, we anticipate changes to succession planning and leadership development related to the use of digital technology, which will support the rapid growth of programs and create a greater network of interconnected information. We have already seen the incorporation of computer-based training, which allows participants to complete a curriculum at a time that is convenient for them and at their own pace. Participants can learn fundamental principles of leadership on their own, allowing coaching and classroom sessions to be more dynamic and interactive.

As our organization expanded geographically, we started to incorporate distance training. Bringing everyone into a single classroom is not always practical or possible, particularly in the case of participants in distant offices who would have a significant commuting burden added to their days of training. By adding screens and cameras both in remote locations and in primary classrooms, individuals can participate in sessions in real time.

We also expect that technology will significantly improve the ability to track the progress of participants in succession planning programs. Many organizations are acquiring succession planning management software, which would allow the Architect, her team, and a participant's coach to communicate electronically with one another. Notes from coaching sessions or classes could easily be recorded and accessed by appropriate individuals on an ongoing basis. The idea is much the same as an electronic medical record system: Key individuals can share information via a single online platform to create a comprehensive file on each participant, simplifying the process for creating a short list of potential candidates when a leadership role becomes available. The Architect would easily be able to obtain the relevant data to determine which participants possess the competencies required to be considered for the position.

We will now take an in-depth look at our retooling of the leadership training program that predated succession planning in our organization, as well as the value that this retooling provided.

OVERHAULING LEADERSHIP TRAINING

After our organization had operated its succession planning program for seven years, we turned a critical eye to enhancing the program, looking for ways to streamline, improve, and refine the leadership development process. Succession planning focused on the development of individuals referred to the program; if the program was to be sustained, we had to move beyond this group and reinforce our commitment to developing leaders throughout the organization. We had a leadership training program in place at the time, but when we examined employees' compliance with the program, we discovered an alarming statistic: In 2013, only 42 percent of our level A–D leaders were engaged in leadership training even though the program was required of all level A–D leaders, not just those who were participants in succession planning.

We investigated the reasons behind this low compliance. Many leaders had started the training but had not completed it; some had been putting the training off for years. Many organizations might have chosen to crack down on their leadership teams, go through a large round of layoffs, and tighten up the requirements for their current program. However, the statistics we were seeing didn't fit the profiles of the leaders we worked with daily. These were people who cared about doing a good job, who were invested in the company, and who believed in its values. We believed strongly in our leadership team's abilities and potential, and we also believed strongly in the training's importance. So why weren't more people completing the program? We took a closer look at the program to find the answer.

IDENTIFYING PROGRAM LIMITATIONS

When the leadership training program was first developed, it was fundamentally based in an educational framework. This mind-set placed high value on the quantity of material transmitted, assuming that the more classes an individual took, the more his competencies would develop. We realized that this approach was not teaching our leaders effectively. We needed to be more sensitive to the time they had for development and make the most of every moment they spent in a classroom setting. Although the classes always had an interactive component, we needed to expand on that aspect so that leaders felt completely engaged with the concepts they were learning and were able to translate those concepts into the realities of their daily on-the-job experiences.

We also recognized that the program had a significant number of redundancies, which meant we were not making the best use of our leaders' time and energy. Many leaders felt they were not able to make the time commitment the program required. They saw their job as their foremost responsibility and didn't have enough room left in their schedules to complete the leadership training as it was currently structured. As we looked ahead to the ongoing expansion of the organization, we also saw we would need tools and strategies to accommodate an ever-increasing number of leaders with a broader range of leadership experience and from dispersed geographical regions.

> I sat in on the entire leadership training and realized it was too much information. We needed to rework the program to be more respectful of our employees' time.
>
> —Steve

RETOOLING THE PROGRAM

Improving the Program Structure and Emphasis

Based on the observations just described, we devised five goals for restructuring our leadership training program. These goals aimed to increase the percentage of leaders who completed the program within the given time limits, both by making the process easier and by emphasizing the importance of leadership development in our organization:

1. Streamline program content to eliminate redundancies and make more effective use of leaders' time.
2. Increase the interactive and experiential aspects of the curriculum.
3. Place the organization's culture and values at the core of the training.
4. Use technology to make learning more effective and to accommodate our broadening geographic area.
5. Make it clear that leadership development is an integral part of each leader's responsibilities as an employee.

After reviewing the curriculum, we found that streamlining the program and eliminating redundancies made leadership training much more manageable. We combined classes that had similar aims; one 16-hour training course on process improvement was streamlined to a single 4-hour class with supplemental computer-based training (CBT) focused on the concepts and tools used in process improvement. We also combined classes on leadership values and coaching because we recognized that their content was similar. Some courses that were previously required because they were considered "core" were made elective; even so, after we revamped the program to make it more relevant and manageable, most participants were eager to take the elective courses anyway.

To emphasize the interactive aspect of the classes, we incorporated more experiential small-group exercises that allowed participants to share their experiences. (These breakout sessions would later provide the model for group coaching.) We encouraged participants to use scenarios and experiences from their own work lives and incorporated role-play to actively engage them. By allowing participants to interact dynamically with the material, we heightened their learning and retention of concepts.

Recognizing that we wanted the leadership training program to establish a firm foundation for our organization's quality culture, we reworked some of the class material as well. As we modified the emphasis of the curriculum, we found that the coursework became more cohesive and more relevant to our unique organizational culture. The curriculum's core classes were all geared toward giving leaders a solid understanding of our cultural values as a company.

To update leadership training through effective use of technology, we began to supplement our classes with CBT, which gave leaders the opportunity to return and review a class's fundamentals. Previously, we had found that by the time leaders got to the program's capstone class, their competence on content from earlier classes had suffered. CBT allowed them to refresh those skills and concepts, leading to increased competence at the end of the program. We also began implementing technology to connect with leaders at our other locations, allowing us to maintain high-quality standards in the classroom while reaching larger numbers of people. (See the discussion earlier in this chapter for more information on the benefits of distance learning.)

Retooling the program allowed us to create a more dynamic classroom experience during leadership training. We even changed our formal assessment at the end, gearing it toward demonstrable skills. Participants must know and understand our quality model, demonstrate skills in conflict management and mediation, and explain how to manage in the face of change. It took about three years to fully shift the program to where we wanted it to be. The iterative process requires patience and plenty of time; some new tactics may succeed, whereas others may take you back to the drawing board. Ultimately, however, we were able to create a program in which the fundamental skills of leadership began to clearly guide the decision-making of our management team.

Clarifying Requirements and Consequences

To achieve the fifth goal (i.e., to make it clear that leadership development is an integral part of each leader's responsibilities as an employee), we needed to find a way to make the training vital not just in theory but also in practice. When we looked closely at the training requirements, we saw that our own guidelines were loose and unstructured. We had made the training a requirement for all leaders but had not provided a due date or deadline. The guidelines never said *when* an individual had to complete the training. Therefore, far too many well-meaning leaders intended to complete their leadership training but never got around to it. Our lack of clarity had led to a lack of initiative among our employees.

Once we realized that we had not clearly defined the structure, we implemented a two-year timeline for completing the leadership training. This timeline was divided into two tracks:

1. If a leader chose to do only the core classes (including the capstone class), the training had to be completed within the first year of hire or promotion.
2. If a leader chose to take additional elective classes (and this was strongly encouraged), the timeline was extended to two years.

We also had to address the fact that noncompliance with leadership training incurred no consequences. The timeline we implemented would help, to be sure, but what would happen if a leader didn't complete the requisite training within one or two years? We needed to add a consequence for noncompliance to improve our results.

Integrating a consequence that has weight without being overly punitive can be tricky, and our particular approach needed to be formulated as a policy endorsed by key leadership. After careful consideration, we opted for a two-tiered consequence. If a leader did not finish her leadership training—either four core classes and a capstone class within the first year or core classes, electives, and capstone class within two years—she received a warning. The next consequence was more serious: If the leader did not complete the training requirement in the following year, she was not eligible for a merit increase until her training was complete.

> Once we told our leaders that they would not be eligible for a merit increase, I had people standing in my doorway saying, "That's not going to happen. How do I register for these classes?"
> —Kathie

This final step demonstrated unequivocally to our team that leadership development was among our company's core values. It also brought us to the point where full compliance for leadership training within two years was the norm rather than the exception. Once our leaders started attending the classes, they saw the benefits of the training and were much more likely to monitor the attendance of their direct reports. New leaders also received clear guidelines for leadership training compliance during their three-day management orientation and started to take initiative on their own to begin the training. Only very rarely did new leaders have to be reminded that their deadline was approaching.

What made the difference? First and foremost, we achieved our goal of making it easier for candidates to complete their leadership training. We eliminated redundancy and waste, made the program more engaging, and tailored the curriculum to be more relevant to our leaders and their jobs. We focused leadership development on our organization's values and quality culture, and we improved remote systems and computer-based learning to accommodate our growing needs across a larger geographic region.

In clarifying the guidelines for the leadership training program, and by instituting a consequence for noncompliance with its requirements, we demonstrated our dedication to leadership development and to the values and skills that are integral to our company's culture. We took a program from a great concept to a substantive commitment in our organization. In doing so, our belief that leadership skills would help us move forward as a company was finally put into practice and has become, as we say, part of our DNA.

As we drew distinct parameters for leadership training, our clarity also helped liberate our leaders. When the guidelines for the program were loose and without a time frame, we were implicitly communicating that leadership training was not a priority. New leaders in the organization may have understood that message to mean that their daily responsibilities carried more weight than completing their leadership training. They might, consciously or subconsciously, push the training to the bottom of their agenda because they wanted to do the best job possible in the areas that they perceived mattered most to us as an organization. Once they understood not only that leadership development was a critical area for the organization but also that this training would expose them to strategies that would enhance their leadership skills, they were free to prioritize it in their schedules, even if that meant temporarily putting less focus on other duties.

We can't emphasize enough that this organization-wide commitment to leadership development starts at the top. Although the Architect is the focus for much of the construction and facilitation of the succession planning and leadership development programs, the Visionary plays a vital and ongoing role in leadership development. His commitment shows support for, and highlights the importance of, the competencies that underscore an organization's culture. The Visionary must be the first to prioritize leadership training, and that includes supporting his direct reports in their commitment to the program.

> I have to be committed to succession planning and leadership development, and my successor has to be committed to it when I retire. People watch everything that the CEO does. When you explain what you want and why it matters, it becomes pretty easy for people to align with what you see.
>
> —Steve

CREATING A SECOND LEADERSHIP TRAINING TRACK

Approximately a year before we decided to overhaul the leadership training program, we added our level E leaders to the program. We soon realized, however, that the program was not adequately meeting the needs of these newer leaders. As leadership development and succession planning matured, we became more aware of the need to reach deeper into the organization to provide training to those individuals who were not yet eligible for the existing leadership programs. The Architect's team set about designing several classes for this level of training. But monitoring revealed that the two levels of leadership training were not sufficiently linked.

As we revised the original leadership training, we also created a second track designed to address the more fundamental needs of individuals new to leadership. This became the standard curriculum for our emerging leaders. We recognized that these leaders needed more emphasis on foundational leadership skills. Creating a new track allowed them to develop at their own pace and, ultimately, to thrive. Three years after creating this curriculum, in the spirit of continual evolution, we decided to add a written examination at the culmination of the program. Passing this exam marks successful completion of the program. A full curriculum of these leadership trainings appears in chapter 22.

CHAPTER 13

Designing the Initial
Development Plan

ONE WAY TO accelerate the embedding of leadership development into the DNA of your organization is by providing leaders with an initial development plan (IDP). The purpose of an IDP is to provide a framework for key leadership elements in the organization, such as attending required training, coaching and developing direct reports, committing to the process of continuous improvement, and selecting an area for personal development. The IDP encourages personal growth from the outset, and it helps foster the growth of others in leadership positions at every level.

Around the same time that we modified our leadership training, we realized we wanted to put a greater emphasis on coaching and leading others because an individual's understanding of any skill deepens by teaching it to another person. The IDP was designed to provide a leader with tools to begin developing his team; after two years, the leader uses the skills he has gained to create a new development plan, which replaces the IDP.

MANAGEMENT ORIENTATION

At BayCare, we chose to provide an IDP to every new leader who completes our three-day management orientation as a way to strengthen the development of our talent pipeline. Many organizations have management orientation that provides the fundamental information leaders need to be able to handle the various processes of leadership. Topics covered typically include risk management, corporate responsibility, and use of the human resources and information technology departments.

In addition to this practical training, however, we offered a module emphasizing the leader's role. This presentation clearly outlined the expectations for leaders in our organization, including the applicable leadership training program, the goal of developing others, and an introduction to the IDP. The training participants included some new hires as well as a great many leaders who had been promoted from within. As soon as they joined our management team, we made it clear that ours was a learning organization and that developing oneself and others was a responsibility built into their job descriptions. We feel that too many organizations miss out on this valuable opportunity to instill in new leaders the importance of leadership development to company culture.

USING THE INITIAL DEVELOPMENT PLAN

The IDP is an integral part of leadership development and should be required for any organizational leadership position (levels A–E in exhibit 4.1). The IDP of leadership development serves a purpose similar to that of the executive development plan (EDP) of succession planning (discussed in chapter 8): It creates a structure and sets a direction for an individual's development and growth.

The IDP comes into play at the outset of any leader's ascendancy to a new position, as soon as management orientation is complete. This immediate deployment not only helps the leader integrate the plan as soon as she begins her new position but also reinforces the importance of leadership development as a core value of the organization.

The IDP is intended to establish the leader's trajectory as she begins her journey in a leadership role and to set the course for her initial growth and development. Thereafter, her boss works with her to create a new development plan. If she is subsequently admitted into the succession planning program, her EDP would be more comprehensive and individualized and would therefore replace her IDP.

INDIVIDUAL DEVELOPMENT PLAN SPECIFICS

The IDP outlines several expectations for the first two years that an individual occupies a leadership role:

- **Leadership development curriculum.** All of our leaders are required to complete the leadership development curriculum within two years. The coursework and timeline are laid out clearly so that new leaders have all the necessary information to schedule and complete the program. Each group of leaders attends the leadership training that is assigned according to their level of leadership (levels A–D and level E; more information about these curricula can be found in chapter 22).
- **Goal of developing others.** Developing others is a goal included in the IDPs of all of our organization's leaders. The requirement to develop others is supported by classes in the leadership development curriculum that focus on values, quality, and coaching skills. We want to cultivate our leaders' mind-set so that they desire to continually improve their methods, rather than abandon what they have learned after they complete their leadership training.
- **Continuous improvement goal.** Continuous process improvement is another expectation we implemented for leaders organization-wide. All newly hired or promoted leaders are required to attend a class (included at all levels of leadership training) focused on understanding process improvement tools; the continuous improvement goal in

the IDP complements this class. Leaders are expected to work with their teams to identify a work process in their area of the organization that would potentially benefit from exploring alternative approaches.

Your organization may use specific tools to monitor the continuous improvement initiatives carried out by employees across the organization. This IDP goal carries a dual benefit in that leaders may choose to identify members of their team who wish to develop skills in the areas of process improvement. As part of their development plans, these team members may be assigned additional classes to enhance their skills and to champion their team's continuous improvement efforts.

- **Personal growth goal.** The last part of the IDP is a personal growth goal. This goal is tailored to the individual and is typically drawn from the leadership competencies used to evaluate individuals in the leadership development program. For this purpose, we recommend that all new leaders take the DiSC assessment prior to attending their management orientation. The DiSC is a behavioral assessment that identifies four categories of intrapersonal tendencies: dominance, influence, steadiness, and conscientiousness. It measures participants' relative strengths in these areas and identifies how the results are likely to be displayed in their roles as leaders. Participants can then receive group feedback on their results during orientation. This assessment leads to an increased understanding of oneself and an understanding of the interplay between a leader's personal behavioral characteristics and those of individuals he may manage. As part of the IDP, a leader would then be asked to choose an aspect of the DiSC that would lead to an enhanced skill, often communication.

By including a personal growth goal in the IDP, we ensured that even leaders who were not in the succession planning program had the opportunity to grow and expand their skills. Once a personal growth goal is identified, the Architect and her team can offer advice and resources for achieving success—for example, attending specific workshops, interacting differently with coworkers, or even implementing an organizational system at work. For newer and younger leaders, the personal growth goal gives a taste of what participating in the succession planning program will be like.

CHAPTER 14

Implementing Group Coaching

AFTER A FEW years, your succession planning program will likely be ready for expansion. At BayCare, we found that within two years of implementing succession planning for our level A–C leaders (as portrayed in exhibit 4.1), we were ready to scale the program. Our primary goal was to create depth in the leadership field to help establish the talent pipeline by which we could boost our company's internal promotions to the desired 80 percent mark. This meant looking beyond established executives, who had been in leadership positions for several years, to younger employees who in many cases were new to their roles. We were now ready to reach our managers at level D.

Based on the increased number of new participants that our leadership development program would now encompass, as well as the resources we currently had available, we determined that one-on-one coaching would not be the best fit for these individuals. Because we had so many level D leaders, we recognized on a practical level that asking their superiors (the level C leaders) to coach them individually would place significant demands on the level C leaders' time. We felt these demands might be considerable enough that they would adversely affect the quality of work that our level C leaders were able to deliver. Therefore, we needed to develop an alternative to coaching our level D leaders as we incorporated them into the succession planning program.

Group coaching, which is an effective way of teaching leadership fundamentals, was the best fit for these newer leaders. Group coaching allowed us to reach a large number of people at once and did not impose a heavy burden on the energy and time of our level C leaders.

Newer leaders tend to have common needs regarding leadership competencies that do not require one-on-one coaching and can be efficiently addressed through group coaching instead. In these group sessions, participants help one another develop the basic competencies of leadership; the group coaching format establishes an environment that creates collaboration among newer leaders across different areas in the organization, rather than fostering a sense of intense competition as candidates jockey for promotions and higher positions.

The interpersonal dynamics of group coaching sessions require a special skill set, because the coach must be able to provide ideas to stimulate discussion and then step back and allow the group to process them, intervening when direction or clarification may be helpful. Initially in our organization, group coaching was done solely by members of the Architect's team. Over time, however, we recognized that there was an additional opportunity to "help leaders lead" by training some of our leaders in effective group coaching. Leaders with a large number of direct reports now facilitate their own group coaching sessions, in some instances.

We use group coaching to address the needs of leaders in two ways:

1. The Architect's team can schedule sessions that focus on a single topic or competency, such as promoting accountability or managing conflict. Leaders can be assigned to attend these group coaching sessions as a way to address competency gaps identified in their development plans, or they may themselves decide to attend a session if the topic is an area in which they wish to grow. The interplay among the members of these

groups offers significant benefits to them. Topic-specific groups may be attended by leaders with varying strengths in that topic, and as leaders share experiences with each another, they also learn from one another. The process of being able to coach a peer enhances a leader's self-concept and also often opens the door for that leader to be more receptive of feedback.

The learning that occurs in this format can be more powerful than that in a facilitator-focused group. The Architect's team becomes proficient at providing structure and a starting point and then allows the leaders in the group to share and respond to one another. An effective group coaching facilitator is like the conductor of an orchestra, bringing out the best performance in each member but not playing each instrument himself. Because having multiple candidates in a session makes the dynamics of group coaching more complicated, we recommend that a member of the Architect's team—one with advanced skills in conflict resolution and group management—facilitate these sessions.

2. Group coaching can be an effective way for leaders in the organization to meet their goal of developing others, particularly if they have a large number of direct reports. In these sessions, the coaching provided would focus on the particular issues and needs of an individual leader's department and the day-to-day activities of her team. Leaders may require some additional training from the Architect's team to learn how to coach for group dynamics.

As your succession planning program continues to grow, you might consider offering one-on-one coaching to all succession planning participants. Alternatively, you could offer one-on-one coaching to your level D leaders in the succession planning program, and then offer group coaching to level D leaders who are not in the succession planning program, particularly if their level C superior has a large number of direct reports. Group coaching works well for many leaders and is a highly effective method under the right circumstances.

CHAPTER 15

Expanding and Differentiating Leadership Tracks

THREE YEARS INTO our succession planning process, we began to expand our reach beyond key leadership. To further develop a foundation for the succession planning program, we established group coaching and began incorporating level D leaders into succession planning, as described in chapter 14.

> A strong leadership development program doesn't need to be built all at once. Start small and then expand as the organization is ready.
>
> —Kathie

We also were ready to establish even more depth in our talent pipeline for future leadership in the organization. We knew we wanted to increase the number of leaders we could help develop. We recognized that operating the succession planning program was an intense process, both for the candidates and for the Architect and her team. We did not believe we could offer a quality assessment experience, feedback, and concentrated coaching for every leader in the organization, nor did we feel that every leader in the organization would necessarily benefit from such a process.

In our talent pipeline, we saw that we could provide a set of fundamental leadership skills (e.g., understanding the impact of change, increasing interpersonal effectiveness, and enhancing communication skills) for a large number of individuals, to help them grow in their leadership competencies. Many of these individuals were new in their leadership careers, and it would be years before they would be prepared for succession planning and key leadership roles in the organization. Adding our level D leaders to succession planning with group coaching was a good beginning, but it didn't ultimately meet all our needs.

To that end, we started to reexamine the leadership curriculum we had in place. We wanted to create training that would meet the needs of leaders at their level of experience and skill, and we also wanted to bring more individuals into the leadership development process. From these goals, we looked at creating tiers of leadership development that were based on individuals' levels of experience. We had already revamped our leadership training and added a second curriculum, as described in chapter 12. We realized that by expanding the program to individuals who were not yet at the management level, hundreds of new, aspiring leaders who were just beginning their careers could be added to the program.

The end product of this examination was three fully differentiated leadership tracks: Experienced Leaders, Emerging Leaders, and Aspiring Leaders (see exhibit 15.1). All three leadership tracks are considered part of the talent pipeline, and for Emerging Leaders and Aspiring Leaders in particular, the leadership competencies are developed without regard to any specific promotion or direction where they may be headed next in the organization.

EXPERIENCED LEADERS

The Experienced Leader track is composed of individuals in level A–D positions. Experienced Leaders are a vital part of the company's talent pipeline and receive many opportunities to expand their skills. Although everyone in your succession planning program will be an Experienced Leader, not all Experienced Leaders will be part of the

Exhibit 15.1: Experienced, Emerging, and Aspiring Leader Tracks

Tier 1

Traditional Succession Planning

Tier 2

Talent Pipeline contains three tracks of leadership development: Experienced, Emerging, and Aspiring.

Experienced Leaders

- Identified by job code; hold a position of executive leadership in the organization
- All succession planning candidates are experienced leaders, but not all experienced leaders are in succession planning

The Experienced Leader track includes the following:

- Leadership certification program
- Coaching (one-on-one, group, and/or informal)
- Development plan to guide growth (initial development plan in first two years)
- Experienced Leaders provide coaching to direct reports as part of their goal to develop others
- Experienced Leaders always go through management orientation, which includes a module on expectations for leaders in the organization

Emerging Leaders

- Identified by job code; hold a position of leadership in the organization
- Newer leaders in the organization; curriculum is a blend of Experienced Leader classes and Aspiring Leader classes

The Emerging Leader track includes the following:

- Leadership training program
- Coaching (one-on-one, group, and/or informal)
- Development plan to guide growth (initial development plan in first two years)
- Emerging Leaders provide coaching to direct reports as part of their goal to develop others
- Emerging Leaders always go through management orientation, which includes a module on expectations for leaders in the organization

Aspiring Leaders

- Individuals who show leadership potential in the organization
- Brought into the program by referral from direct superior

The Aspiring Leader track includes the following:

- Aspiring Leader curriculum
- Coaching (one-on-one, group, and/or informal)

succession planning program. The leadership training requirement described below is based on a leader's position in the organization and is applicable whether or not that leader is a participant in succession planning.

The Experienced Leader curriculum includes the leadership certification program. Experienced Leaders who are also in succession planning will receive one-on-one coaching, and those not in succession planning may receive either one-on-one or group coaching, depending on the number of direct reports their boss is expected to coach. After completing management orientation, each new leader receives an initial development plan (IDP), as described in chapter 13. If an Experienced Leader is in the succession planning program, his executive development plan will replace his IDP. Experienced Leaders provide coaching to their own direct reports as part of their goal of developing others. Supplemental workshops, training, and mentorship may also be part of their leadership development, although these resources are primarily allocated to Experienced Leaders who are also in the succession planning program.

EMERGING LEADERS

Participation in the Emerging Leader track is determined by an individual's job code. The Emerging Leader track is composed of level E candidates and includes roles such as supervisors and assistant managers. Although these individuals are responsible for leading people, they are just beginning their leadership careers. As such, they receive training across a broad framework of leadership concepts.

The Emerging Leader training includes a required leadership training curriculum that is a blend of classes from the Experienced Leaders and Aspiring Leaders curricula. (A sample of these classes appears in chapter 22.) These classes are to be completed within two years of hire or promotion into an Emerging Leader position. Emerging Leaders receive an IDP after completing management orientation as well as coaching, because their bosses are Experienced Leaders who have the goal of developing others as part of their development plan. Emerging Leaders are expected to provide coaching to their direct reports because they, too, have the goal of developing others as part of their IDP. Because Emerging Leaders tend to have a large number of direct reports, coaching usually takes place in group-facilitated or informal on-the-job settings.

ASPIRING LEADERS

The Aspiring Leader track is for individuals who do not yet hold leadership positions in the company, but who show leadership potential. Of all the tracks, Aspiring Leaders probably do the most to distinguish themselves to their superiors, because they are identified solely by their performance on the job.

The Aspiring Leader training includes a course curriculum designed specifically for the development needs of this population (see chapter 22 for a sample). Because of the cascading effect of leadership development and the goal of developing others that all leaders have, a leader who refers an individual to the Aspiring Leader program commits to providing coaching to help that individual internalize the material presented in the classes.

Adding the Aspiring Leader track was a significant contribution to the longevity of the organization.

—Larry

Our Aspiring Leader program currently has more than 500 participants and is continually growing. Some of our most rewarding work has been with these individuals, because they are so enthusiastic about growing and learning new skills.

—Kathie

Look at the impact that 500 Aspiring Leaders have on the culture of our company. We've been able to do so much in the past ten years; imagine what we will have achieved ten years down the road. When I think about how inspired these individuals are and where they're going, I see that they're going to make a huge difference to the future of our organization.

—Steve

As leaders ascend in an organization, their leadership track may change. Once an Aspiring Leader becomes an Emerging Leader, for example, she is required to complete additional classes as part of her leadership training. She will not, however, have to repeat any courses she has already taken as part of the Aspiring Leader curriculum.

IDENTIFYING TEAM MEMBERS WITH LEADERSHIP POTENTIAL

One aim of leadership coaching is to instill the practice of always being on the lookout for nascent leadership abilities in team members throughout the organization:

- An employee who is always up for a new challenge, who identifies ways to get things done effectively and efficiently, is likely a creative thinker.
- An employee who volunteers to lead a project, drawing others into both supporting the process and taking pride in their accomplishments, is likely a leader of people.
- An employee who comes to you with an idea for accomplishing a recurring process in a more cost-effective way is likely someone with financial acumen worth developing.

In these instances and others like them, it behooves those in leadership positions to have an "antenna of potential" and to look beyond the mere accomplishment of daily assignments. This level of awareness in leadership befits an organization that has a long-term view of development. Acknowledging employees' nascent leadership characteristics has the potential to strengthen the commitment of those individuals to the organization.

CASE STUDY

A manager in human resources established development plans with each of her direct reports. During regular quarterly meetings to review progress, she noticed that one of her direct reports approached these review sessions in an extremely organized manner, sharing a summary of the progress she had made on her goals and providing a list of topics for discussion. Beyond her investment in her own professional development, this employee also used her review sessions to share ideas she had for changes to processes that would potentially enhance the quality of the services the team provided. This capacity to think beyond herself and to have a broader, departmental view indicated that this individual had nascent potential to move into a leadership position. To support this potential, the manager referred her to the Aspiring Leader program so that she could refine her skills and take her potential to the next level.

CREATING LEADERSHIP TRACKS FOR DISTINCT POPULATIONS

Generally, you want to do your best to integrate the entire population of your organization into a single leadership development program. Although candidates eventually may be placed into different tracks based on their experience and competencies, the content of each track should be structured to contain a common language while providing different levels of leadership competencies. This practice strengthens the idea that leadership development is a part of the organization from top to bottom and gives younger leaders the chance to model and learn from leaders in more senior positions.

Your organization may have a distinct population that doesn't easily fit into the overall succession planning and leadership development trajectory. In our case, as we started to look at the future of healthcare and where we thought BayCare was headed, we determined that physicians were going to play a larger administrative and executive role in the company. We wanted to give them the leadership skills they would need to play that part effectively, but after trying to integrate them into our standard leadership development model, we found that it was more effective to train physicians in the specific competencies that their roles required. We realized we needed an ancillary program specific to them.

A physician's day-to-day job is distinct from that of an executive or administrator. Furthermore, physicians were not likely to be in the same pool for succession planning as the rest of our leadership team; we did not anticipate that a physician would ascend to a position such as chief financial officer or senior vice president of operations. Therefore, we created a leadership track specifically for physicians, one that places a much greater emphasis on a specialty focus—in this case, healthcare.

When designing the training, we also considered the necessary accommodations for physicians' unusual and demanding schedules, and we needed to be certain that our program complied with state laws concerning the kind of training and resources we could legally provide to physicians. We also sought to offer this population the opportunity to fulfill some of their CME (continuing medical education) requirements where appropriate.

In seeking to provide physicians with the competencies they needed to become effective leaders, we created a program that focused on elements of leading teams; handling conflict openly and fairly; managing the change process by leading through it rather than mandating it; and offering strategies for building trust, communicating effectively, and demonstrating personal accountability. The physician leadership training also included an introduction to financial basics, managed care fundamentals, and strategic thinking. The program was formatted according to the perspective of physicians, using their language and examples from the patient care world, to concretize their learning.

SHOULD EVERYONE LEARN TO LEAD?

Following is an all-too-common scenario for an organization that lacks the infrastructure of a supportive leadership development program.

Suppose you have a fantastic employee. He is by far the best X-ray technician in your company. He interacts with patients in a professional and reassuring way, documents all care encounters thoroughly, and can be relied on to include the needed anatomy in all of the diagnostic scans he performs. When the level E leader position of supervisor in the X-ray department becomes available, it seems logical to promote this X-ray technician to the role, despite his lack of leadership experience.

The X-ray technician finds that as a supervisor, he suddenly has to spend far more time on administrative responsibilities than before. In fact, he takes hardly any X-rays at all, which is the work that he really loves. He feels unequipped to manage his team of people because he doesn't know much about leadership. He can't help but interfere when he sees his employees doing things that he could do better. He starts micromanaging his staff and neglects his administrative role. As the performance of the X-ray department begins to decline, the new supervisor is quickly pulled from his leadership role and is replaced.

What happened here? Clearly, just because someone excels at a job does not guarantee he will excel at managing others who do the same job. Although the supervisor in this story needs to have a thorough working knowledge of X-rays, the best person for the job also has a vested interest in leading others. This particular X-ray technician is happier taking X-rays all day, and although he is likely to appreciate a higher salary, his promotion ultimately left him feeling less satisfied with the prospect of going to work each morning.

The first important lesson from this example is that individuals in leadership positions are most successful when they have the desire to lead. The second lesson is that organizations without strong leadership development programs do not have the resources to help their employees when difficult situations arise. If a strong program had been in place, the organization might have first attempted to nurture the X-ray technician's leadership abilities, rather than immediately terminate him. If this individual was interested in leading the department but felt he lacked leadership ability, he could be offered coaching to help strengthen his leadership competencies. Alternatively, his boss or a member of the Architect's team might have worked with him at the outset in a supportive environment and determined that the X-ray technician was not well suited to a leadership role. The organization would then look to place him where he could be most effective, rather than allow him to struggle in a situation where his career was potentially at stake.

In the leadership development program that we have been describing throughout this book, the X-ray technician-turned-manager would have immediately gone through a three-day management orientation and received an IDP. He would have been placed in the Emerging Leader track, taken classes in the leadership training curriculum, and received one-on-one coaching by his boss or in an informal setting. These measures would have made him much more likely to lead his department successfully.

Creating a Leadership Development Team

WE HAVE MADE numerous references throughout this book to the Architect's team, which she ideally will be able to hire as the succession planning program and leadership development training gain ground, provide viable internal candidates, and start to demonstrate cost savings by making expensive external searches unnecessary.

We recommend that all new members of the Architect's team hold a master's degree, primarily because it demonstrates a high level of commitment, substance, and professionalism. Standout individuals with only a bachelor's degree may be considered for entry-level positions. Ideal candidates will have a background in organizational development, executive coaching, psychology, education, or a combination thereof. Of course, there are exceptions; as with any hiring process, sometimes "gut instinct" factors into a hiring decision.

Members of the Architect's team must be eager and willing to learn because they will likely pursue continuing education, such as an executive coaching certification, while on the job. They need outstanding communication skills because they will be working closely with participants in the leadership development and succession planning programs. They will also need to have presence and a dynamic personality to create an exciting and engaging environment when they facilitate group coaching sessions and leadership development classes.

Even though these individuals may not technically hold leadership positions in the company in a traditional sense, they are leaders to all program participants with whom they work. Therefore, each team member needs to display strong leadership characteristics and be actively involved in the leadership training classes, whether for Experienced, Emerging, or Aspiring Leaders. Furthermore, when working with succession planning program participants, these leadership coaches will be administering and interpreting assessments, creating executive development plans, and providing feedback and coaching.

At BayCare, we built a team of four leadership coaches who taught all of the courses in the leadership development curricula and worked with leaders who were referred to the succession planning program. The work of these coaches often overlaps with that of individuals in the classroom and subsequently in succession planning. Their role is labor-intensive because they not only are teaching workshops that are one and a half to two days long but are also providing individual feedback to participants in many classes, such as those on managing conflict or the capstone assessment class. These leadership coaches must be passionate about the material, love working with people, and be committed to helping others grow.

When your organization is ready to expand the Architect's team, it is best to keep these positions separate from the human resources department. Even though both teams deal with interpersonal conflict and professional growth, human resources should remain outside the realm of succession planning and leadership development to avoid the potential for conflicts of interest. Candidates who fail to participate meaningfully in the programs may be dismissed from the succession planning program, but this should in no way affect the security of the position they hold in the company. Separating human resources from the Architect's team helps ensure neutrality for your human resources department and gives the Architect's team the freedom to provide feedback and guidance openly to participants in the succession planning program and individuals in the leadership tracks.

COACHING METHODS: DIRECTIVE FACILITATION

In addition to offering members of the Architect's team the opportunity to become certified executive leadership coaches, our employees were all trained in-house on the Directive Facilitation Model coauthored by our very own Architect, Dr. Kathie Dies, in collaboration with Dr. Robert R. Dies (see exhibit 16.1). These 21 principles for effective coaching originally started in the psychology world as

---

Exhibit 16.1: Directive Facilitation

Develop a realistic contract.

I nstill a positive climate.

R eact with a process rather than a person focus.

E mploy a proactive coaching style.

C ounter obstacles to professional development.

T ranslate conflict and resistance.

I llustrate your theory of change.

V alidate the importance of feedback.

E ncourage employee responsibility.

F acilitate a here-and-now focus.

A ctivate a search for common themes.

C onfront troublesome behaviors.

I nclude sharing strategies for continued development.

L ead employee into behavioral practice.

I ntegrate professional development and team strategic goals.

T ie together work experiences.

A ct as a conduit for expanded experiences through collaboration.

T urn attention to unfinished development.

I nitiate opportunities for peer coaching.

O penly encourage the sharing of competencies and learning from others.

N urture the personal and professional growth of those who report to you.

---

principles of group psychotherapy, but their application to coaching has been a tremendous boon to the field. In our organization, the concepts frame how we think about providing coaching and are introduced to our leaders as they learn how to coach. Each letter highlights a different aspect of coaching theory and methodology:

- **Develop a realistic contract.** The coach should work closely with the individual to establish a development plan that reflects opportunities for growth. The coach should also be committed to providing guidance and meaningful opportunities to both enhance the participant's current competencies and explore new areas for professional growth.
- **Instill a positive climate.** Coaching is intended to create a safe environment for growth and development. Acknowledging and building on the candidate's current strengths to provide the foundation for growth is an effective way to instill a positive climate.
- **React with a process rather than people focus.** The coach should focus on the process of demonstrating competencies, not on the personality of the individual. Even when the participant's personality traits are very much at play, this should be cast in the light of the behaviors and characteristics that are necessary to lead effectively.
- **Employ a proactive coaching style.** A proactive coach is on the lookout for ways to enrich the participant's development. Although the key responsibility to seek coaching is on the shoulders of the participant, a proactive leader considers the candidate's development goals and is vigilant in identifying competency-expanding opportunities.
- **Counter obstacles to professional development.** When a participant experiences an obstacle to learning or enhancing a competency, it is the role of the coach to seek

ways to counter that obstacle and find alternative paths to achieve the development goals. For example, suppose a participant has taken on a new responsibility that precludes her from attending a workshop that would help her become more proficient in a competency area. The coach can either structure one-on-one time to discuss the topic covered by the workshop or rearrange staff coverage to enable the participant to attend it.

- **Translate conflict and resistance.** A coach must be capable of differentiating between resistance and a lack of understanding. When a participant fails to make expected progress toward a development goal, the first step is to examine the goal to make certain it accurately reflects her desired growth. Perceived resistance and conflict may be the surface behavior of some underlying issue that is blocking her progress. A response that takes a "help me understand" approach can open the door for her to share otherwise unknown concerns, fears, or uncertainties that may be blocking progress. Once these issues come into the open, the coach is in a better position to help her move forward effectively.

- **Illustrate your theory of change.** In many instances, the coaching process involves helping the participant recognize the behavioral changes required to demonstrate increased competency. A coach needs to provide a framework for understanding why the change is important. For example, the coach may draw a parallel between the participant's own struggles with behavioral change and the challenges his team encounters when faced with changing processes. The candidate may react with denial as he struggles to see why the behavioral change is important. The coach engages with the participant to assist him in moving beyond this resistance to change by helping him see the benefit to his professional growth and increased competency. The skills the coach uses are similar to those the participant will need as he works with his own team members to help them recognize the personal benefits a process change might bring. Once resistance is overcome, the behavioral change process can move on to active learning, where the participant is given opportunities to both learn and practice acquired leadership skills. During this time, the coach highlights the importance of providing both knowledge and skills acquisition for the participant's team during times of change. The final stage of illustrating a theory of change occurs when the coach provides reinforcement. A coach who is tuned in to the benefits of positive feedback is more likely to facilitate the participant's ongoing professional growth and development.

- **Validate the importance of feedback.** As the coach works with the participant to integrate feedback, a key component of the coach's role is to validate why this feedback is important and how it plays into the participant's overall personal and professional growth.

- **Encourage employee responsibility.** It is easy for a participant to lean on the coach for all aspects of the process. However, the coach is not there to motivate but rather to inspire the desire for development. Each participant is expected to be accountable for his own development process, articulating his needs and initiating action steps himself rather than waiting for the coach to take the lead.

- **Facilitate a here-and-now focus.** Often during a coaching session, the participant demonstrates the exact behaviors that have been identified as needing adjustment. For example, a participant may be striving to demonstrate more active listening when talking with her direct reports, and in the context of coaching she stops listening so that she can plan what to say next. The coach can bring this here-and-now example into play, removing the need to talk in the hypothetical.

- **Activate a search for common themes.** This practice can occur in both individual and group coaching. In individual coaching, the coach may provide a participant with feedback about a competency as viewed by various individuals the participant works with; the feedback's common themes make it difficult for the participant to dismiss the feedback. In group coaching, highlighting common themes among members of the group opens the door for broader exploration of the group dynamic.
- **Confront troublesome behaviors.** Sugarcoating and avoidance have no place in the coaching arena. An effective coach confronts troublesome behaviors in an open and honest manner, maintaining a respectful demeanor while addressing the need for change.
- **Include sharing strategies for continued development.** A coach who also is working on personal and professional development not only talks the talk but also walks the walk. Sharing experiences of growth, and of struggles with growth, can be an amazingly powerful component of the coaching process. However, be prudent when sharing any negative struggles. Too negative an experience can have just the opposite effect and alienate the participant from the coaching process.
- **Lead employee into behavioral practice.** Coaching sessions are great starting points for professional growth because discussions can lead to increased understanding. However, to concretize skills, participants equally need opportunities to practice them.
- **Integrate professional development and team strategic goals.** When a coach is able to connect the individual participant's development goals with the accomplishment of a team goal, obvious benefits accrue to all concerned.

For example, providing a participant with the opportunity to lead a strategic key project can develop his skills while meeting the team's goal.

- **Tie together work experiences.** The coaching experience is a time for the coach to help connect the dots between the participant's daily work experiences and the goals on the development plan. When the daily tasks toward a goal can be matched to an identified growth opportunity, the coaching becomes a dual win.

- **Act as a conduit for expanded experiences through collaboration.** A coach can encourage growth through expanded experiences. Sometimes the coach can facilitate those experiences by assigning tasks that require the development of additional skills. Other times, the coach uses her connections throughout the organization to facilitate the individual's involvement in a project with another team, or in a job-sharing experience where the development of two individuals can be enhanced through collaboration.

- **Turn attention to unfinished development.** Coaches give development assignments, monitor progress, and provide feedback. Although they expect the individuals they are coaching to demonstrate personal accountability for development, they provide guidance to keep development on track until completion or adjust development plans to best address the need for additional competencies.

- **Initiate opportunities for peer coaching.** One of the most impactful approaches to professional development is for a coach to lead her team in peer coaching. By identifying the unique strengths and growth opportunities of each member of the team, an effective coach can link together peers who mutually benefit by sharing their areas of expertise with one another. Often, the learning that is experienced with a peer has a greater impact than that experienced with the coach.

- **Openly encourage the sharing of competencies and learning from others.** The more the coach encourages her team members to share their development plans with one another, the greater the opportunity for peer coaching. One of the most effective practices is for the coach herself to be transparent enough to share her own development goals, thereby reinforcing her commitment to creating a learning environment for her team.
- **Nurture the personal and professional growth of those who report to you.** A leader's commitment to coach her direct reports in their professional growth requires the capacity to communicate expectations clearly, to listen carefully to the needs and motivations of those she is coaching, to treat errors as learning opportunities, and to reinforce the mediating steps that ultimately lead to the achievement of goals. In doing so, she creates a fertile ground in which the seeds of development can be nurtured to full growth.

CHAPTER 17

Creating a Team of Coaches

COACHING THE COACHES

As we have mentioned, most candidates in the succession planning program will have their direct superior assigned as their coach. This arrangement serves two purposes: (1) It helps the coaches learn and fully integrate leadership skills by teaching them to somebody else, and (2) it allows an organization to scale the leadership development program successfully. To help our leaders learn to coach others, we found it necessary to provide all organization leaders with mandatory training in the art of coaching. Using a newly created computer-based training (CBT) program, the training provided a basic framework and strategies for coaching others. Additionally, a class focused on developing coaching skills that reflect organizational values was revamped to provide strategies and practice to help new leaders start off successfully with their coaching competencies. Finally, the CBT and class were often supplemented with one-on-one sessions to "coach the coaches."

Depending on the size of the organization, this process will require time to develop. Some coaches will voluntarily reach out for sessions to improve their skills, whereas human resources or team member surveys may be needed to identify other coaches who require additional skills work to enhance their coaching abilities.

All leaders who have direct reports are expected to provide development opportunities and coaching to their reports. Leaders who do not have direct reports may be encouraged to provide mentoring to junior leaders to strengthen their skills. This policy goes hand in hand with the goal of developing others that is assigned to all individuals in leadership positions. Even leaders who are not in the succession planning program are expected to coach their direct reports, and the resources to improve coaching competencies are available to all organization leaders.

> Every individual in an organization can benefit not only from receiving coaching but also from being a coach.
>
> —Kathie

The coaching sessions are guided by the individual being coached, with the expectation that candidates will bring questions, problems, and issues for discussion. Both the coach and the Architect's team are responsible for making this expectation clear, particularly if a candidate has never worked under a coaching modality before. Initially, coaching is based on the candidate's initial development plan (IDP), but it likely will

CASE STUDY

A hospital executive in a large healthcare system was particularly adept at mentoring his direct reports. Key leadership and the Architect's team recognized his skills on a number of occasions. When the time came for more formal coaching in the organization, he was asked to help identify other leaders who demonstrated effective coaching skills in their individual teams. A list of these individuals was then circulated to all organization leaders, who were invited to reach out to them for guidance when leadership development questions arose.

evolve over time as the candidate's proficiency increases or as he is assigned additional responsibilities that require a new or enhanced skill set. Coaching sessions can grow out of something the candidate has experienced while carrying out her daily tasks, an area she would like to explore to better understand a strategic initiative, or a desire to expand her industry knowledge base.

COACHING AND LEADERSHIP TRACKS

Coaching is a dynamic, flowing process in which the candidate and coach work together to craft the unique learning experiences that make up a participant's development. A coach's role is to listen, reinforce, challenge respectfully, provide resources, and monitor growth.

Whereas a candidate's leadership track (Experienced, Emerging, or Aspiring) is based on either his job code (for Experienced and Emerging Leaders) or referral to the program (for Aspiring Leaders), the kind of coaching the candidate receives is based on a much more fluid structure. If your organization expects all leaders to provide coaching for their teams, and if your organization makes it a high priority to promote growth for all leaders, you will likely need to give your managers a high degree of autonomy when determining the best way to coach their direct reports. A leader who has a small team of employees will probably offer one-on-one coaching. With a larger team, one-on-one coaching becomes more prohibitive, and the primary format will likely need to be group coaching where the leader can address common elements of professional growth for many individuals at once.

For example, a level D leader with 40 direct reports would be hard-pressed to provide 40 private coaching sessions every quarter. In this case, the leader could identify the most motivated members of his team and prioritize their coaching, while ensuring that other employees receive informal coaching on the job and all the training they need to do their jobs effectively. Logically, then, an Aspiring Leader who is one of the level D leader's direct reports would be prioritized to receive coaching; the level D leader would readily identify the Aspiring Leader's potential, having been the person who referred him to the program in the first place.

Note that although we are talking about participants in leadership tracks *receiving* coaching, the imperative is on the leaders who are *providing* the coaching. This is another reason we recommend allowing leaders to structure the way they choose to coach their direct reports: It is part of the leader's development plan first, and part of the leadership tracks for those receiving coaching second. (Again, one exception is the succession planning program, which is separate from the leadership tracks and offers one-on-one coaching for all participants at levels A–D.)

SETTING AND HOLDING BOUNDARIES

A coach should understand her personal limitations and notify the Architect's team if she is having difficulty in sessions with an individual or if she has concerns about an individual's health and safety because of information revealed during coaching sessions. The organization may determine that covering the costs of outside support for certain employees is a worthwhile investment. If that determination is made, coaches will benefit from knowing that additional resources are available to assist in clarifying a participant's ultimate needs and who can best help the participant access those additional resources.

In such matters, strong collaboration between the Architect's team and the human resources department is vital. Both entities should be available as resources for a coach who has concerns that go beyond the boundaries of a coaching relationship. Partnering with human resources is important to ensure you are complying with any laws and regulations about how such referrals should be handled. Additionally, the Architect's team may be able to use these circumstances as a teaching moment for the coach, helping him through the process of seeking additional resources and appropriately supporting the participant in need of assistance.

STRATEGIES FOR EFFECTIVE COACHING

The desire to see others grow and develop is the foundation for effective coaching. Only then can there be the kind of connection that fosters such growth. That being said, the following strategies can enhance one's coaching skills:

- Cascade the expectation of coaching direct reports throughout the organization.
- Provide hesitant coaches with support as they develop their skills to coach their direct reports effectively.
- Follow Directive Facilitation principles (see chapter 16) through the stages of forming, storming, norming, and performing (Tuckman 1965) in the coaching relationship.
- Encourage coaches to seek an understanding of the individual's strengths and identify learning opportunities through assessment tools or explorative conversation.
- Monitor the ongoing measurement and reshaping of development goals throughout the cascading process of coaching.
- Identify mentors who can both help coaches gain additional skills and supplement coaching experiences by providing expertise in disciplines outside the coaches' areas.

Some organizations recognize effective coaches in the ranks of leadership and capitalize on their skills to educate others in the coaching process. Other organizations consult an outside coach to establish training to be carried out by new or existing team members. Whatever the approach, a cascading coaching process is the key to ongoing success in developing internal talent.

CASE STUDY

While launching a succession planning program, one organization identified the cascading coaching model as one of the pillars on which to build the program. To this end, an executive coach was added to the organizational structure to develop a coaching program and train a team of coaches to promote effective coaching among leaders beyond the executive level. New coaching classes were designed, and attendance was a required part of every new leader's onboarding process. One-on-one mentoring was put in place, and all IDPs for new leaders contained the goal of developing others. A copy of this IDP was sent to each leader's superior as a mechanism for monitoring the individual's goals and progress. The elements of this approach—a team of coaches who worked with the Architect, a structured program to train leaders to coach their direct reports, and the written expectation that leaders must develop others—emphasized the organization's commitment to the succession planning process.

REFERENCE

Tuckman, B. W. 1965. "Developmental Sequence in Small Groups." *Psychological Bulletin* 63 (6): 384–99.

CHAPTER 18

Fostering Commitment and Collaboration

LEADERSHIP DEVELOPMENT DOES not happen in a vacuum. Leaders need the support of the entire organization to achieve the most favorable outcomes possible, and the support of the leader's boss is critical to success.

In chapter 6, we discussed the reasons we recommend that managers refer candidates to the succession planning program and the Aspiring Leader track of leadership development (Experienced and Emerging Leaders always receive leadership development based on their roles in the organization). When a candidate is referred to succession planning, a full assessment battery is completed, and the results are integrated with those from any other assessments done during management orientation and leadership training. All of this data is considered when drafting the participant's executive development plan (EDP). The individual is enrolled in (or will have already completed) leadership training and establishes a coaching relationship with his boss.

A candidate referred to the Aspiring Leader track follows the course curriculum for that level of development. If the referring manager has not yet established a coaching relationship with the participant, a member of the Architect's team will ask her to do so. Our policy is that the candidate's boss must support the candidate's participation in the program, for two reasons:

1. The manager is accountable for ensuring the candidate's responsibilities are covered during the time he misses work because of the curriculum. Changing the schedule, revising project timelines, and reassigning duties to other employees may strain a department, and the manager is in a better position to recognize this situation than members of the Architect's team are. The Architect and her team want to work in consort with the boss to create a positive learning environment with the least amount of disruption to the candidate's routine responsibilities. Succession planning participants are at a high level in the organization, so they are not as vulnerable to disruption as, say, individuals in the Aspiring Leader track, such as leaders of customer-facing areas or employees whose primary responsibility is to deliver services. In the case of Aspiring Leaders, class attendance or coaching sessions may require that responsibilities be redistributed across an entire team.

2. The boss is a significant link in the candidate's support chain. The boss is expected to support the candidate's growth and development through a variety of training resources, to make growth opportunities available through role sharing or role expansion, and to provide coaching. Together, they work through issues that the candidate faces daily in the workplace. By respecting managers' authority, and by having solicited referrals from them previously, you automatically co-opt them into the succession planning and leadership development processes. Doing so fosters an environment of support and camaraderie between manager and candidate.

   The manager's support is particularly important for Aspiring Leader track participants. These individuals are not yet in leadership positions; according to their job descriptions, they are responsible for the direct provision of services. As such, managers need to be mindful of the

Aspiring Leader program's expectations and be willing to accommodate the time necessary for their direct reports to receive this training. Aspiring Leaders are in the program because their managers recommended them, which signals that the managers have committed to their development. In fact, our referral form for Aspiring Leaders requires the recommending manager's signature, with a statement that reads, "I support the time necessary for this individual to be developed."

> Our leadership team was not on board in this way a decade ago. Now when I ask their permission for participants to attend workshops and courses, the answer is almost always, "Yes, of course! What a wonderful opportunity." The participant doesn't go on the roster until I hear back from the manager, and that speaks to the kind of contract that exists between the two parties. Once they have both agreed to the training, there exists a mutual accountability for class attendance and follow-through.
>
> —Kathie

Under these circumstances, only rarely does a manager turn down a participant's request to take time off for leadership training. When it does happen, it signifies that in addition to developing the participant, you may need to offer the manager some direct coaching, too. The mind-set "I can't afford to let this person go" does not accord with the aims of a learning organization; you can't be a learning organization without building learning opportunities into your structure. Employees in the program receive both leadership development and on-the-job training, whatever their role. We strive to bring those two pieces as closely together as possible so that what participants learn in one role can be directly applied in another. This alignment is cost-efficient, makes employees more effective, and helps embed a culture of learning and leadership development into the fabric of the organization.

CREATE TIME AND SPACE TO COACH DIRECT REPORTS

In their roles as coaches, members of the leadership team not only need to allow participants to take time off work for leadership training but also must create time in their own schedules to develop those participants. Often the participants' coaching is informal and focuses on dealing with issues as they arise in the workplace. Pairing coaches with their direct reports creates plenty of opportunities for this kind of interaction. However, we also recommend asking coaches to schedule one formal quarterly session with participants—dedicated time when the participant has the coach's full attention and can ask questions and introduce topics that may require deeper discussion.

In chapter 5, we mentioned the cascading effect of succession planning. As your employees see an increase in internal promotions in the levels of leadership above them, their mind-set shifts to one of opportunity and possibility. This phenomenon is top-down and starts with the CEO. The process of creating time for formal coaching is similar; it is a reverse cascade effect that starts from the bottom of an organization and moves upward. If a manager makes time in his schedule to coach his direct reports, then *his* manager must understand that some of his resources are diverted for that purpose, *her* manager must also understand, and so forth. This is one more reason it is vital to integrate an approach of internal development into the company's DNA.

IT STARTS WITH THE VISIONARY

The Visionary continues to play an active part in the succession planning and leadership development processes. He should have individuals in succession planning whom he coaches directly, and he should be required to complete the same certification process as every other leader in the company. Making exceptions for those in higher office conveys a sense of elitism and runs completely counter to the egalitarian culture of opportunity that you are trying to create. We can't stress it enough: Regardless of how beautifully constructed your program is, succession planning and leadership development programs will succeed only if you have a Visionary who supports those programs with his actions every single day.

> The CEO has to be the biggest supporter of succession planning and leadership development for it to work. He or she should be highly involved in the process on an ongoing basis.
>
> —Steve

SUCCESSION PLANNING CONSIDERATIONS

Because a referral to the succession planning program starts with a candid conversation between a boss and her direct report, we have seldom encountered a candidate who is reluctant to participate in the program. We have, however, regularly heard candidates ask certain questions about the program. The Architect can address these questions during the structured interview that is part of the initial succession planning process. The following are some of the questions most frequently asked:

- **What happens if I do poorly on the assessment battery?** Sometimes a candidate fears that a "negative" result on the assessment battery will be detrimental to her career. If she voices this concern, the Architect can clarify that the assessment battery is not used to rule anybody out of succession planning. Rather, it is used to identify where and how the EDP can be structured to best support and nurture the candidate's leadership abilities. Once a candidate's boss has made the referral and the candidate herself is prepared to commit to the program, the organization reciprocates by committing to the candidate's growth and development.

- **What if I am not interested in a promotion?** Occasionally, a candidate feels comfortable in his current role and is not necessarily looking to be promoted. In such cases, we always position the succession planning referral as a way to improve the candidate's competencies on a day-to-day basis, leaving the option open for a change of heart about promotion in the future. When a candidate realizes he can be even better at what he currently does, he is often highly motivated and excels in the program.

- **Once I am part of succession planning, you will see all my competency gaps. Will this put me at a disadvantage when I'm compared with external candidates for a position?** When the Architect hears this question, she can first emphasize that the organization does not directly pit internal candidates against external candidates (see chapter 10). Additionally, external candidates often take many of the same assessments as internal candidates, and their assessment results are available to any organization that is considering hiring them. Thus, the internal candidate is actually at an advantage because the organization has information not only about her gaps but also about her progress in closing those gaps over time. This kind of ongoing data is not typically available for external candidates.

- **What if I don't succeed in the program?** The answer to this question depends on how the candidate defines success. Some individuals do not grow in the succession planning program, largely because they do not take advantage of the coaching, training, and other opportunities made available to them. Pointing out to these individuals that they may be passed over for promotions is often sufficient motivation to increase their commitment to the program and to their personal development goals.

The most important question the Architect can ask a new candidate is "What does being referred to succession planning mean to you?" The candidate's answer will allow you to clearly see the level of commitment he is bringing to the program, as well as to correct any misconceptions he may have. At the outset of our program, we had some individuals who wanted to participate because it seemed like an honor and an advantage; however, they were not prepared to commit to the work that was necessary to succeed. We redirected the efforts of most of these individuals through coaching, but for a few individuals succession planning was simply not the right fit.

If a succession planning program offers such advantages, wouldn't putting all your leaders into the program be beneficial? The short answer is no. On the one hand, we want all our leaders to grow, and we want their direct reports to grow as well. On the other hand, we do not wish to place an undue burden on any individual who may have extenuating circumstances or who is not interested in moving into a larger leadership role. Furthermore, at a certain point, incorporating all your leaders into a succession planning program simply isn't feasible. The number of candidates and the amount of resources required would far outweigh the number of available positions in the organization, and the program would no longer be practical. This is why we recommend keeping the more focused and intense succession planning an optional, referral-based program. You want to entice those individuals who are interested and excited about participating, while still requiring all leaders to be part of the leadership development process.

CHAPTER 19

Measuring Success

ONCE SUCCESSION PLANNING is under way, it is only natural that the Visionary, the Architect, and especially the board will want to see some measure of the program's success. Ideally, you conveyed to your board from the outset that succession planning is a long-term strategy; two or three years into the program, however, you may be asked to defend your position.

A succession planning program needs five to seven years to mature (possibly longer, if you are rolling out new phases during that period). This time frame allows you to collect adequate information to ascertain whether any internal candidates are ready to assume key leadership roles. You also need at least this amount of time to gather sufficient data about replacing leaders with internal candidates versus external ones. Remember, for the first few years of succession planning, you may still be hiring external candidates most of the time. Only after five years did our organization have enough data to significantly increase our hiring of internal candidates for key leadership roles.

The data you collect comes primarily from the program participants' coaches. The Architect's team checks in with the coaches on a regular basis (typically once a year, although software technology may enable a more real-time process). This coaching review provides a sense of the participants' growth and development. The Architect's team keeps notes in each participant's file that will be consulted when participants are considered for a short list of prospects for a newly vacant position in the company.

SETTING THE CRITERIA FOR SUCCESS

The most valuable step you can take when measuring the impact of a succession planning program is to set clear criteria for determining its success. These criteria should be decided early on, during the planning phase of program implementation. Here are four specific criteria for success that can be applied to your organization:

1. **An increased percentage of leadership positions are filled by internal candidates.** Perhaps the most obvious measure of success, and the one we have been discussing throughout this book, is a shift in the percentage of leadership positions that are filled by internal candidates as opposed to external ones. For our company, it felt right to take a 20-to-80 ratio of hiring internal versus external candidates and to flip those numbers. After a decade of succession planning, we had achieved an approximately 75-to-25 ratio, which we consider an immense success. Your organization may have different target numbers, and your shift may be more or less dramatic than ours. What's important, however, is setting a clear goal rather than just looking for a general increase in the number of internal candidates who are promoted. Setting a clear target helps you strengthen the culture around succession planning, because you can rally the entire company around a specific aim. It also helps you present measurable statistics to both your employees and your board.

    Keep in mind that this shift in percentage is an outcome—a sign that your succession planning program is working effectively. Your main focus should remain on the process itself, streamlining and refining the program until it runs as smoothly as possible. You are seeking to promote only the best candidates into higher leadership roles. If you continually experience an insufficient number of internal candidates to keep the process competitive, you will need to identify which areas of the organization are underrepresented and remind the leaders of those areas that developing the competency of their teams is a top organizational priority. If you are confident in the training that you offer your leaders, you must ensure there is a matching commitment to training across the organization. The message of this top-down approach to succession planning is that all leaders are personally accountable for developing the employees in their areas so that the organization has the greatest opportunity to promote from within whenever possible.

2. **Candidates in the program improve their competencies.** Another clear measure of success on a granular level is that candidates show progress in developing their competencies. In fact, this may be the most important factor in determining the success of a succession planning program: If the candidates do not demonstrate personal growth, they likely won't be qualified to ascend to higher positions in the organization, and the percentage of external-to-internal hires likely won't shift significantly.

   What might progress look like? Suppose a candidate needs assistance in developing her financial acumen, which her initial assessments may have identified as a weakness or which she needs to develop for a future role in the company. Whatever the reason, the candidate has difficulty integrating and analyzing financial data. She takes classes and workshops that specifically target financial skills. Since she is already working in finance, she is assigned a mentor in that department. After undergoing this specialized training, she is asked to create a forecast for her department. Whereas her previous forecasts were not accurate, she is now within the expected margin, showing that she has improved her skills, has a solid grasp of financial concepts, and can now forecast for her department effectively.

3. **Leadership development is fully integrated into the organization's DNA.** Occasionally, the measure of success cannot be quantified but instead appears when you realize that the ideas of leadership development have crystallized in the organization. At BayCare, we have made developing others a high priority for all our leaders. In the following box, our Architect describes the day she watched one leader teach another about this concept.

I was in a meeting where we were proposing development plans, and we were trying to get a group of leaders on board with us. One leader said, "Well, I'm going to be selfish here. If my direct report has time for development, there are other things I need her to do." Another piped up and said, "No, no, no, you don't understand. Your *job* is developing your direct report." I felt comfortable enough to set a date for retirement after that conversation, because I saw that some leaders really got it and could carry on the goals of the program.

—Kathie

---

4. **The company has adopted a mind-set of "look inside first."** One of the most obvious changes we have observed as a result of succession planning occurs during management orientation. This three-day training is the first touch point between the Architect's team and a newly hired leader. As you would expect from a successful leadership development program, we see large numbers of people who have been promoted from within. The mind-set has shifted so much in our company that internal candidates are automatically considered first. We have also seen a number of level D leaders who are not participants

in succession planning but who are nonetheless promoted to level C positions; the organizational mind-set has become sufficiently pervasive that internal candidates at this level are automatically considered for these roles. The biggest impact of the program has been this 180-degree flip in positioning from a 20-to-80 split to almost the reverse.

Another huge accomplishment of the succession planning program is that our board became internally focused. A company's board always returns to the lens of representing the community. For a public company, of course, the community is the shareholders. Boards view their job as ensuring that their organization's resources are used as effectively as possible. They do not necessarily feel obligated to scour the world looking for the best candidate to fill a role, nor are they necessarily committed to developing the employees who already work for their company.

We were able to show our board that having an individual's development plan alongside his experience provides more information about him than an external candidate's curriculum vitae does. We demonstrated that promoting from within makes more sense on a community level, that giving employees more opportunities means better retention, and that supporting internal growth builds on the investment of employees who deeply care about the organization. This approach is now so ingrained that the board calls BayCare a "succession planning company."

METRICS OF MEASUREMENT

Leadership development metrics encompass as wide a range of statistics as the organization chooses to consider. These metrics can range from individual improvement on development plan goals to the percentage of internal versus external hires for leadership positions, the number of degrees or certifications achieved, or the impact on recruitment costs and onboarding time. Here are examples of metrics in specific program areas:

- **Succession planning.** At the beginning of the program, take an assessment of key leadership hires over the course of the previous five years, the percentage of internal versus external hires, the cost of recruiting externally, and the cost of downtime associated with bringing external hires up to speed with the organization's direction and culture. Chart the progress in these areas across the years, preferably in an annual report to the board.
- **Talent management.** Establish, via a human resources tracking system, the development goals of individuals in the program and measure how those goals are achieved. A straightforward, easily measured goal would be whether an individual completed a degree or training certificate. A less straightforward goal (measuring a "softer" skill) would be improved interpersonal communication. Monitor feedback on annual reviews as a way of gathering viable statistics for goals relating to softer skills.
- **Leadership development.** An organization may have a specific training course that all leaders are expected to complete as part of their initial development process. Track how many leaders complete this course.

CASE STUDY

In BayCare's succession planning program, the metrics covered two levels: organizational and individual. The organizational measures were assigned costs in dollars and time. Tracking the balance of internal versus external hires into leadership roles and

→

---

the financial impact of recruiting, onboarding, and downtime as new leaders acclimated to their roles demonstrated that hiring internal candidates was less expensive. For example, the cost of recruiting a president to lead all hospital operations throughout the system was eliminated by hiring from among qualified internal candidates who were already fully familiar with the BayCare quality culture and operational processes.

Individual metrics for participants in the succession planning program were less concrete but could be measured by administering an initial assessment battery (see chapter 7) and then tracking progress on the goals that grew out of the assessments. Such goals included completing assigned classes, achieving a degree, receiving positive feedback from peers, or successfully advancing the professional development of direct reports. Review of these metrics created a readiness report that indicated whether any internal candidates could be considered for leadership vacancies in the organization.

SUCCESS REQUIRES CONSEQUENCES

As we learned from our own experience with leadership training, creating a beautifully structured program and getting your leaders to complete it are two different matters. Success is measured less by great ideas and more by compliance with and consistent execution of those great ideas. As explained in chapter 12, we recommend establishing a clear time frame for completing any required certifications or programs, which allows your candidates the freedom to fulfill the requirements at their own pace while still taking care of their day-to-day responsibilities. In addition to establishing a deadline, you must also implement a consequence for noncompliance. Otherwise, employees will think, "I didn't complete the program on time. So what?" The consequence you choose sends a clear message about the importance of leadership development in your organization. A significant consequence, such as not allowing leaders to be eligible for a merit increase unless their leadership training is completed within the specified time frame, demonstrates that leadership development is vital to your company. It also speaks to the value that you place on employees' integrity. You are conveying that they are accountable for following through on their commitments, and this accountability must be consistent throughout the organization, from the CEO on down.

> The best way for the Board Advocate to be in the loop is for the Architect to provide the board with regular progress reports on the succession planning and leadership development programs.
> —Larry

IS IT CONSIDERED A SUCCESS IF EXECUTIVES LEAVE?

Many organizations look at succession planning and implicitly place a numeric value on each executive in the program. They see individuals as being "worth" the training and resources that have been invested in their development. When an executive chooses to leave the organization, this numeric value is then viewed as a loss to the company, a poor investment, or a failure.

The reality is that executives will (and sometimes should) depart even the healthiest and most nurturing of organizations. A company may prepare three executives to assume the CEO's role even though, in the end, only one will actually ascend to the position. The leaders who were not promoted may find that their expanded competencies now allow them to change organizations, perhaps even becoming CEOs somewhere else.

I remember reading about Jack Welch, CEO of GE, and the way he nurtured four of his top leaders to replace him. Once he selected a successor, the other candidates all left the organization to become CEOs of Fortune 500 companies. I heard people in the business world suggest that the training and investment he put into those candidates was a waste of time and money, but I felt just the opposite. While those individuals were part of GE, Jack Welch had four CEO-caliber executives working for him. That's the real gift of succession planning—working with immensely capable and skilled individuals, even if for a short while. Those executives were great leaders who no doubt inspired their employees, most of whom are still with GE. You can't underestimate the value of having fantastic executives working for you.

—Steve

In an organization with relatively few tiers of leadership positions, you must assume that you will develop some leaders who ultimately will leave your company. Their timeline for promotion and the timing of key leadership openings may simply not coincide. Just as an organization should not promise a position to any leader in advance, leaders are not obligated to promise career-long dedication to a company that is offering to develop their skills. If you can learn to value these leaders for what they offer while they are part of your organization, you will feel a sense of pride and accomplishment when they depart because you contributed to their professional development. You may even find that you can create partnerships with other organizations through the experiences they gained working with you. Exhibit 19.1 shows how many leaders have participated in BayCare's succession planning program and talent pipeline, as well as how many have stayed and left.

Exhibit 19.1: Succession Planning by the Numbers

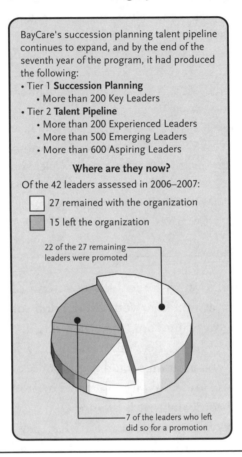

BayCare's succession planning talent pipeline continues to expand, and by the end of the seventh year of the program, it had produced the following:

- Tier 1 **Succession Planning**
  - More than 200 Key Leaders
- Tier 2 **Talent Pipeline**
  - More than 200 Experienced Leaders
  - More than 500 Emerging Leaders
  - More than 600 Aspiring Leaders

Where are they now?

Of the 42 leaders assessed in 2006–2007:

27 remained with the organization

15 left the organization

22 of the 27 remaining leaders were promoted

7 of the leaders who left did so for a promotion

MILLENNIALS: CONSIDERING A NEW GENERATION

Will your succession planning program continue to be successful as a younger generation—the millennials—rises through the ranks? Is the leadership development process time-tested enough that it can cross generational lines and be sustainable in the future? These are the kinds of questions that far-thinking Visionaries all over the country should be asking themselves today.

Certainly the best-researched generation to date, millennials and what they are looking for in the workplace have been the main focus of numerous articles and studies. Meister and Willyerd (2010) put it succinctly: Millennials want "a constant stream of feedback" and are "in a hurry for success." They also prize mentoring and coaching and consider leadership one of the top five skills they want to learn on the job.

This "constant stream of feedback" means that millennials want to be recognized for their competencies. The structures of succession planning and leadership development allow for exactly that by defining measurable skills and abilities and allowing individuals to track their progress over time. The coaching and mentoring elements of succession planning and leadership development programs also offer this generation the opportunity to solicit advice, receive critique, and learn from their elders in a way they seem to crave.

The "in a hurry for success" aspect of the millennial mind-set is a bit more problematic. An organization may find that if it can't provide the internal resources for young leaders to grow and develop at the pace they prefer, then it is likely to lose some of these individuals to opportunities outside of the organization—which is one more reason to start succession planning and leadership development sooner rather than later. The more strongly your company emphasizes internal promotion, the greater the chance it will meet the needs of a swiftly moving generation and turn those individuals into long-term employees.

Structuring curricula and courses for these "digital natives" may also require revising certain aspects of succession planning and leadership development programs. In the future, you may want to offer candidates the option to complete some of their coursework online or on a work-from-home basis. We began to address this need by using computer-based training to provide foundational knowledge, maximizing the amount of time in the classroom devoted to the application of learning. Organizations should already be including topics such as ethics in the social media space in their leadership and conflict resolution training.

Even if the rising generation possesses unique characteristics, we believe that the basic models of succession planning and leadership development are fundamentally aligned with the concepts and practices that are necessary to strengthen the culture of any organization: fostering the growth of current employees, cultivating a culture that looks inside first, and keeping costs down while you do it. The framework of a succession planning and leadership development model may look very different a decade from now, but we expect that the fundamental principles on which it is built will remain just as strong.

REFERENCE

Meister, J. C., and K. Willyerd. 2010. "Mentoring Millennials." *Harvard Business Review*. Published May. https://hbr.org/2010/05/mentoring-millennials.

CHAPTER 20

Putting It Together

LET'S LOOK AT an example of the way succession planning is intended to cascade through an organization. It begins with the announced retirement of a level B leader, a division vice president.

The level B leader approaches the Architect approximately three years after the start of the succession planning program. This leader is forward-thinking and has determined that his retirement is about five years away. He himself is not a participant in succession planning, but he has referred three of his level C direct reports to the program and has asked for guidance in coaching each of them to prepare for possibly replacing him when he retires. (As an aside, one of the individuals he referred had moved to her level C role by previously accepting two lateral promotions, which helped expand her experience base before making a ladder move.)

Over the next five years, these three individuals are not only coached but also given expanded roles to broaden their experience bases. They are encouraged to attend national conferences, and all of them reach a level where they are presenting at conferences as well. Whenever one of them has a significant accomplishment, the division vice president contacts the Architect so that the achievement can be noted in the candidate's succession planning file. As the division vice president works with each of his direct reports, he provides valuable ongoing feedback on their professional growth.

By the time he retires, he is able to clearly identify and recommend the most qualified individual to succeed him.

Because of the critical nature of the division in the organization, his recommended successor is given the promotion on an interim basis. Her coaching continues in her new reporting structure, and four months later, she is officially awarded the level B role. While she is in the role in an interim capacity, an external candidate search for the position is not conducted, demonstrating the organization's support for her.

The transition doesn't end there. When the new level B leader officially moves into her role, she promotes one of her former peers into the level C role she just vacated. This promotion is a lateral move that is intended to broaden that individual's experience base. This cross-promotion opens another level C position, and although an internal level D leader applies, the new division vice president decides that this internal candidate is not the best fit. She chooses to conduct an external search and hires someone from outside the organization for this level C role.

Within a year, it becomes clear that the external hire is not a good fit for the organization's culture. At that point, the level D leader who had previously applied is promoted to the role on an interim basis and is officially confirmed as director within four months. She subsequently recommends one of her direct reports, a participant in the Aspiring Leader program, for promotion to her former managerial role.

The process that unfolded in this example results in four distinct internal promotions: three ladder moves and one lateral move. A level C leader moved to a level B role, a level D leader moved into a level C role, an Aspiring Leader moved into a level D role, and another level C leader was cross-promoted to broaden her experience base. This hypothetical example included some course-corrections, which accurately reflect the process as organic, evolving, and not always linear. For an individual occupying an interim position in such transitions, the Architect should provide additional coaching to enhance the individual's competency base to take advantage of the opportunity to move into a new role. A visual representation of our hypothetical scenario, as well as a general timeline of our recommendations for adopting succession planning and leadership development programs, are shown in exhibits 20.1 and 20.2.

Exhibit 20.1: How Succession Planning Cascades Through Internal Promotions

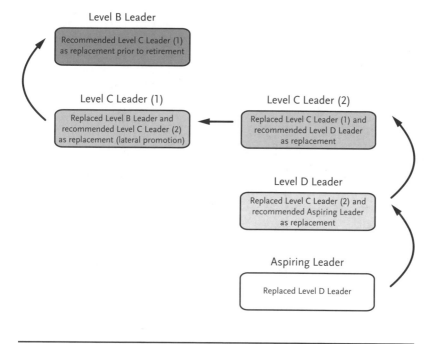

Exhibit 20.2: Timeline of Succession Planning and Leadership Development Implementation

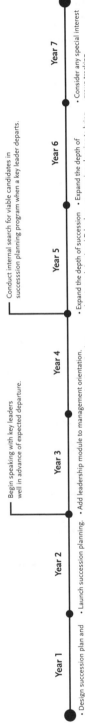

Begin speaking with key leaders well in advance of expected departure.

Conduct internal search for viable candidates in succession planning program when a key leader departs.

Year 1
- Design succession plan and obtain approval from the board.
- Identify key leadership competencies for leaders in your organization.

Year 2
- Launch succession planning.
- Identify process to bring candidates into the program.
- Create format for executive development plans.
- Provide guidelines for coaching.

Year 3
- Add leadership module to management orientation.
- Incorporate initial development plans for all new leaders in the organization.
- Explore ways to expand succession planning to address organizational strategic initiatives.

Year 4

Year 5
- Expand the depth of succession planning to bring Level D leaders into the program.
- Expand the Architect's team to address the growing size of the program.
- Develop the process to be used to identify internal candidates for key leadership roles.
- Expand the coaching program to incorporate group coaching.
- Consider replacing key leaders with internally developed candidates.
- Start to identify and analyze data for progress and potential areas for improvement as the program matures.

Year 6
- Expand the depth of succession planning to bring the most entry-level leaders (Aspiring Leaders) into the program.

Year 7
- Consider any special interest group tracking.
- Develop a process for continual review of competencies, and maintain alignment with organizational strategic initiatives.

Ongoing
- Refine and evaluate the processes in place.
- Review and redefine role descriptions for key leadership positions in the organization.
- Make succession planning a regular item on the board's agenda.

ADDITIONAL RESOURCES

The scope of this book is intentionally a deep dive into one organization's implementation of succession planning and leadership development programs. Readers interested in learning about other organizations' methodologies and case studies may be interested in the following additional resources:

Bennis, W., and R. Townsend. 1995. *Reinventing Leadership: Strategies to Empower the Organization.* New York: William Morrow and Company.

Berke, D. 2005. *Succession Planning and Management: A Guide to Organizational Systems and Practices.* Greensboro, NC: Center for Creative Leadership.

Collins, J. 2011. *How the Mighty Fall: And Why Some Companies Never Give In.* New York: Harper Collins.

Rothwell, W. 2010. *Effective Succession Planning: Ensuring Leadership Continuity and Building Talent from Within,* 4th ed. New York: American Management Association.

Tichy, N. M., and S. Sherman. 1993. *Control Your Destiny or Someone Else Will.* New York: Knopf Doubleday.

Timms, M. 2016. *Succession Planning That Works: The Critical Path of Leadership Development.* Victoria, BC: FriesenPress.

PART V

Nuts and Bolts

CHAPTER 21

Candidate Assessments

As discussed in chapter 7, the assessment battery that succession planning candidates take should encompass intrapersonal skills, interpersonal skills, and emotional intelligence to assess the softer skills of leadership. A 360-degree survey should also be included to target the harder skills of leadership that your organization determines to be paramount to its success, such as strategic planning or financial acumen.

Numerous assessments are available on the market, and your Architect can help you choose assessments that are specific to your organization. Some tests are considered industry standards, and the Architect may have personal experience with certain assessments as well. Ultimately, however, the values, skills, and competencies tested by the assessment battery should align with your organization's values and goals so that the assessments provide truly meaningful feedback. In this chapter, we describe the assessments we recommend.

DiSC ASSESSMENT

The DiSC assessment (www.discprofile.com), discussed in chapter 13, is a standard assessment that measures interpersonal skills according to four behavior traits: dominance, influence, steadiness, and conscientiousness. We recommend that all leaders take this assessment as part of management orientation or similar programs. The DiSC report may be included in the results from the succession planning assessment battery as an additional source of data. DiSC assessment data can also be incorporated into several classes in the leadership development curricula and used to provide information to help shape the personal growth goal in a leader's initial development plan.

MYERS-BRIGGS TYPE INDICATOR

An industry standard in assessment, the Myers-Briggs Type Indicator (MBTI; www.myersbriggs.org/my-mbti-personality-type) helps leaders identify their preferences along four continuums. By understanding their preferences, leaders are better equipped when they are placed in positions that require them to act outside their comfort zones. Type preferences can be described with an analogy: Although you may walk through all the rooms of your home, there are some rooms in which you feel most comfortable. These most comfortable rooms represent your type preferences.

CONFLICT DYNAMICS PROFILE

The Conflict Dynamics Profile (CDP; www.conflictdynamics.org) is one of our favorite examinations. Developed at Eckerd College, the CDP focuses on conflict management and resolution in the workplace. The CDP-I, a self-reporting individual assessment, can be used in the Aspiring Leader and Emerging Leader curricula to help new leaders identify the dynamics of their own reactions to conflict. For Experienced Leaders, you can use the CDP-360, which solicits feedback from the participant, the participant's boss and direct reports, and others. This allows Experienced Leaders to compare their own assessment of how they approach conflict with the perceptions of those around them.

In addition to taking the CDP-360, each Experienced Leader is video recorded while handling conflict in a provided scenario. Then the participant and a member of the Architect's team review the recording to reinforce the participant's demonstration of positive skills or to identify areas in which the participant needs to grow. Thus, the CDP allows you to provide training that matches the participant's level of leadership.

FIRO-BUSINESS

The Myers-Briggs Fundamental Interpersonal Relations Orientation (FIRO) instrument (www.themyersbriggs.com/firo) uses a matrix of needs and wants to measure a candidate's communication skills and relationships with others. The FIRO assessment has two types, FIRO-B and FIRO Business; we prefer the FIRO Business test because it puts the feedback from the FIRO assessment into a report that is geared specifically to business settings, making it more applicable to succession planning. The report examines the candidate's interpersonal characteristics and indicates how these characteristics might play out in interactions with a boss, direct reports, and peers; when negotiating; or in problem solving.

EMOTIONAL INTELLIGENCE

Although a number of emotional intelligence assessments are available, we prefer to measure emotional intelligence in the context of a structured interview. We feel that the yes-or-no format of many emotional intelligence examinations does not portray a candidate's motivations and intentions clearly enough. By integrating emotional intelligence questions directly into a face-to-face interaction, one can gain a much deeper understanding of an individual. Sample questions you might use in an interview include the following:

- How do you respond to situations that are fraught with conflict?
- How do you deal with situations that are full of turmoil?
- How do you maintain a positive, focused attitude when you encounter obstacles to achieving a goal?

LEADERSHIP MIRROR

We recommend the Leadership Mirror assessment from DDI (www.ddiworld.com) for creating a 360-degree feedback survey in the succession planning program. This assessment should not be confused with other 360-degree surveys that your organization may offer its employees, such as those often used in conjunction with annual reviews. All 360-degree assessments solicit input from the candidate; the candidate's boss, direct reports, and peers; and others in the organization who may not be direct reports or peers but still have a valued perspective on the leader's competencies.

The Leadership Mirror allows you to provide feedback on how a candidate's self-perception aligns with or differs from the perceptions of other groups, as well as on how the perceptions of the various groups providing input differ from one another. For example, a candidate's boss and direct reports might have perspectives that differ from those of peers and others. Exploring the underlying dynamics of these differing perspectives can be a unique learning opportunity for the candidate.

Identifying the competencies to be measured is key when selecting the best 360-degree survey for a given organization. Customizing the competencies allows the assessment to directly reflect the organization's strategic initiatives and to measure its pivotal skills for achieving its goals.

Competencies assessed through the Leadership Mirror can change depending on an organization's strategic initiatives. The most useful Leadership Mirror will contain a mix of hard and soft competencies, as in the following example:

- Adaptability
- Building organizational talent
- Building partnerships
- Building self-insight
- Coaching and developing others
- Compelling communication
- Continuous improvement
- Courage
- Driving execution
- Driving innovation
- Earning trust
- Emotional intelligence essentials
- Empowerment and delegation
- Executive disposition
- Financial acumen
- Influencing
- Leading change
- Leading teams
- Navigating complexity
- Operational decision-making
- Personal growth orientation
- Positive disposition
- Selling the vision

IS REASSESSMENT NECESSARY?

As a rule, we do not recommend administering these examinations more than once. In the first iteration of our succession planning program, we reassessed participants after three years in the program to gauge their progress and growth. We compared the data from the second tests against the feedback we had received directly from the participants' coaches and the notes we had gathered over the past three years. The coaches' evaluations closely matched the growth we saw when the participants retook the assessments. Hence, we determined that administering the tests repeatedly was an unnecessary expense. Our coaches not only had the best insight into the growth of the participants but also were able to point to concrete internal examples that supported their opinions.

> The battery of candidate assessments should be comprehensive and reflect the values of the individual organization.
>
> —Kathie

Course Curricula for Leadership Development

THE CORE CURRICULA for a participant in leadership development will be determined by his or her leadership track: Experienced,
Emerging, or Aspiring. In this chapter, we provide sample curricula
for each leadership track. These courses can be taught by the Architect's team in-house, and each class can be offered several times a
year to ensure leaders are able to complete their requirements within
the specified time frames.

The class size for courses in the Experienced Leaders curriculum
should be capped at 25 participants; these higher-level courses deal
with greater complexities of leadership that are best addressed in a
smaller group setting. The courses in the Aspiring Leader curriculum,
on the other hand, can be taught to approximately 75 participants.
In these classes, experienced facilitators can skillfully split the participants into smaller "breakout" sessions, allowing them to integrate
content effectively while still offering leadership development to
large numbers of people.

EXPERIENCED LEADERS

All Experienced Leaders (levels A–D in our model; see exhibit 4.1)
are required to complete their specific leadership curriculum, which

we refer to at BayCare and in this book as *leadership certification*. The curriculum comprises four core classes; three elective classes on managing conflict, change, and mediation; and a capstone course that measures competency in the skills taught throughout the classes. If a leader takes only the core classes, leadership certification must be completed within the first year of hire or promotion. Leaders who choose to add the electives, which are strongly recommended, are given an additional year to complete the classes before completing their capstone class.

As described in chapter 13, all current leaders are also assigned the goal of developing others as part of the initial development plan that is given to all leaders when they complete management orientation, immediately after hire or promotion to a leadership role.

Sample Experienced Leader Curriculum

Core Classes
    Coaching with the Values
    Role Models for Quality
    Understanding Process Improvement Tools
    When Mistakes Happen: Learning from Our Errors

Elective Classes
    Change Management
    Mediating Workplace Conflict
    Respond to Conflict Effectively

Capstone Class
    Leadership Profile

EMERGING LEADERS

Determined by job code, the Emerging Leader track is for individuals who are newer to leadership positions and are working on developing the skills and competencies required in their current roles. These candidates are in the leadership development program and typically hold level E positions, such as those of supervisor or assistant manager. Emerging Leaders are required to complete all seven classes of their leadership curriculum and to take a final exam that assesses their knowledge after coursework is completed. Four of the courses in the Emerging Leader curriculum are also included in the Aspiring Leader curriculum; participants need to complete these courses only once, so an individual who completed them as part of the Aspiring Leader track does not need to repeat them if promoted to an Emerging Leader role. Similarly, the other three courses are included in the Experienced Leader curriculum, so Emerging Leaders will not need to retake them if later promoted to an Experienced Leader role. Leadership training for Emerging Leaders is expected to be completed within two years.

Sample Emerging Leader Curriculum*

> Coaching with the Values
> Understanding Process Improvement Tools
> When Mistakes Happen: Learning from Our Errors
> First Steps in Managing Conflict
> Foundations for Quality
> Leading a Diverse Workforce
> Navigating Change

*This curriculum includes a written examination once coursework is complete.

ASPIRING LEADERS

Aspiring Leaders do not yet hold leadership positions in the organization, but they have been identified as possessing leadership potential. The curriculum for Aspiring Leaders is designed to meet their unique circumstances of not yet being leaders. By referral to this track, these individuals are exposed to the basics of leadership in preparation for an eventual promotion to a leadership role. As previously mentioned, some Aspiring Leader courses overlap with coursework in the Emerging Leader track. The Aspiring Leader curriculum does not need to be completed within any specified time frame.

Sample Aspiring Leader Curriculum

First Steps in Managing Conflict
Foundations for Quality
Leading a Diverse Workforce
Navigating Change
Coaching
DiSC Strategies
Writing for Results

SUCCESSION PLANNING

As explained earlier, all candidates in succession planning will be Experienced Leaders who have completed the leadership certification. Every succession planning participant will have an individualized executive development plan (EDP) based on the results of the comprehensive assessment battery conducted when the candidate was referred to the program. This EDP includes development goals and growth strategies, one-on-one coaching, and possibly also mentorship in the organization, as well as external resources such as conferences, workshops, and reading assignments. Candidates in this track may be given expanded responsibilities and cross-training in other departments or skills.

SUPPLEMENTAL RESOURCES

BayCare was thrilled to partner with a major state university to create a leadership series designed specifically for participants in our succession planning program. This additional training looks at leadership through a wide lens and includes topics such as innovation and creativity, strategic thinking and planning, financial acumen, driving execution, talent management, emotional intelligence, and executive presentation.

Each module of the training was paired with an action learning project, which participants create and work on in small teams over a period of six months. At the end of the six-month training mode, they present their projects to the organization's level A leaders (the senior leadership team). We have found the skills and competencies taught in these courses to be incredibly beneficial to succession planning participants.

In addition to partnering with a third party to develop auxiliary in-house training, you can send executives to leadership conferences, bring in keynote speakers, host workshops, and engage in team-building exercises. The cost of outside resources can add up quickly, particularly if you factor in expenses such as travel and hotel accommodations, so use these resources only as a supplement to strong in-house competency development.

Conclusion

OUR AIM IN writing this book was single-minded: to show how important succession planning and leadership development are to a healthy, enduring organization. Whether you choose to follow every recommendation in these pages or opt to create a unique program for your company, we believe this book provides the foundational elements for building a solid succession planning program and for creating a talent pipeline to support that program for years to come.

A "culture of leadership" is one of many business concepts that receive universal praise and support, and much lip service has been paid to the notion of an "organization of leaders." The reality, however, is that developing such a culture and organization takes dedication and wholehearted commitment to the process, from the CEO on down. Sound bites and speeches can briefly inspire employees, but they have lasting effects only when paired with solid infrastructure and ongoing education. Just as the Visionary and the Architect are both critical to succession planning and leadership development, so too are the twin pillars of inspiration and infrastructure, each playing a distinct but vital role in the process.

Witnessing our leaders grow and develop, seeing our employees recognize the potential for leadership in themselves, and observing the teaching moments that occur when they share that potential with others have been some of the most rewarding experiences of our careers. Succession planning and leadership development have far-reaching consequences that extend well beyond the organization; our employees take their abilities into their personal lives, sharing them with their families and their communities. It is an honor to think we have contributed to their growth in some small way.

Index

About the Authors

Stephen R. Mason, LFACHE, has dedicated his entire professional career to the health and well-being of others. In his four decades of service in healthcare, Mr. Mason has held several management and leadership roles, most recently as CEO of BayCare Health System, one of the largest regional health systems in the country. As the leader of a company with more than 26,000 employees, he has extensive experience as a "messenger-in-chief," using engaging language and storytelling to distill a message into its simplest form.

His leadership style blends personal experience, soft skills such as effective communication and relationship building, and a commitment to tangible outcomes and measurable improvements. Now retired, Mr. Mason is spending his "second career" pursuing several new ventures, including a role as founding partner of CSuite Solutions, which is helping health systems evolve and adapt to the changing demands of healthcare. He lives with his wife, Wanda, in Washington State.

Mr. Mason served as CEO of BayCare, as chief operating officer and senior executive vice president of Texas Health Resources Inc., as president of Harris Methodist Hospitals, as senior vice president of operations for Hospital Management Professionals Inc., and in hospital administration roles in Kansas and Wisconsin. He served as chairman of the Florida Hospital Association, the United Way of Tampa Bay, the quality committee of Premier Inc., and Tampa Bay Partnership. He has a master's in health administration from the

University of Minnesota and a bachelor's in business administration from Golden Gate University in San Francisco.

Kathryn G. Dies, PhD, is a clinical and sport psychologist with four decades of experience in both private practice and hospital administration. Dr. Dies, alongside her husband, Dr. Robert Dies, developed a theory in the early 1990s based on 21 Principles of Leadership in Psychotherapy Groups and provided training nationally and internationally on these principles. Subsequently, Dr. Dies drew on these principles to shape Directive Facilitation, her approach to effective leadership in working teams. Incorporating aspects of clinical and sport psychology, she bases her approach on the foundation of interpersonal relatedness and motivation for goal achievement.

Working with Mr. Mason, Dr. Dies used her years of experience as an executive coach to develop a comprehensive succession planning program for BayCare Health System. This program is based on an assessment to identify each participant's foundational leadership skills, establishes an individualized development plan, coaches the achievement of goals to fill gaps in leadership skills, measures participants' progress, and creates layers of leadership readiness to address ever-changing organizational needs.

Dr. Dies has a PhD in clinical and community psychology from the University of Maryland. She has worked clinically in outpatient and inpatient settings and with emerging, professional, and Olympic athletes. While providing psychological assessments for Dominion Hospital, a large psychiatric hospital in northern Virginia, Dr. Dies was recruited to join the administrative team to establish a cost-effective assessment program. Promoted to associate administrator, she built a comprehensive partial hospitalization program as a discharge option for patients and their physicians. Her final role with Dominion Hospital was vice president of clinical services. After relocating to Florida, Dr. Dies served as chief operating officer of a Pasco County–based Charter psychiatric hospital before joining BayCare in 1998.

Larry Morgan is the chairman of Morgan Family Ventures, a high-growth group of companies spanning multiple industries.

From humble beginnings on a farm in northeastern Missouri, Mr. Morgan worked his way to and through the University of Missouri, where he graduated with a bachelor's in business administration. After graduating, he served in and was honorably discharged from the US Army and accepted a position with the Firestone Tire & Rubber Company, where he flourished until 1972. For the next 18 years, Mr. Morgan built a small, 7-store tire dealership into a 137-store chain. In 1990 he developed his own tire company, Tires Plus. Within ten years, Mr. Morgan expanded his business to 603 locations in multiple states. He was inducted as a member of the Tire Industry Association's Hall of Fame in 2008. He also served as president of the Tire Industry Association.

In 2000, Mr. Morgan sold his Tires Plus business and began dabbling in the automotive industry with a 50 percent interest in a dual Honda/Volkswagen dealership. Embracing this industry, Mr. Morgan began building his automotive empire with the purchase of Toyota of Tampa Bay in 2005. To date, he has amassed 32 franchised dealerships under the Morgan Auto Group umbrella, with dealership locations stretching across the state of Florida. Highly recognized in the automotive industry, Mr. Morgan was named Florida's 2009 TIME Dealer of the Year by the Florida Automobile Dealers Association. His stores have been separately honored, as well, for their individual positive performance.

Morgan Family Ventures also owns Morgan Construction Management Services, a building contractor; Beth Ingram & Associates Inc. and Integrity Therapy Solutions, both large therapy providers; Compark 75, a warehouse and office commerce park; Creative Sign Designs Inc.; and HR Hernando LLP, a real estate holding entity. Mr. Morgan serves as a member of the board of directors of USAmeriBank and is a board member of SunTrust Bank of Tampa Bay. He has been honored by the *Tampa Bay CEO Magazine* as CEO of the Year and among its 100 Most Influential Business Leaders. In 2004, he was inducted into the Tampa Business Hall of Fame; in 2012, he received the Golden Flame of Philanthropy Award; and in 2014, he won the prestigious Entrepreneur of the Year award.

Mr. Morgan takes an active part in his community and is past chairman of the board of BayCare Health System; the Florida Automobile Dealers Association; and Morton Plant Mease Health Care, to which he also contributed $6 million to build the new Morgan Heart Hospital. He is also a member of the board of the Florida Council on Economic Education; past chairman of the Valspar Championship, the annual PGA golf tournament played at Innisbrook each year for the benefit of area charities; and a member of the Pasco Economic Development Commission.